JUN - - 2011

allergic girl

*adventures in living well
with food allergies*

sloane miller

WILEY

John Wiley & Sons, Inc.

Published by John Wiley & Sons, Inc., Hoboken, New Jersey
Published simultaneously in Canada

Worry-Free Dinners® is a registered trademark of Allergic Girl Resources, Inc.
Allergic Girl® is a registered trademark of Allergic Girl Resources, Inc.

"Kiss On My List," page 102, by Janna Allen and Daryl Hall © 1981 Primary Wave Brian (Janna Sp. Acct.) (BMI) admin. by Wixen Music Publishing, Inc., and Unichappell o/o/ Itself and for Hot Cha Music, all rights reserved, used by permission; *Selected Odes of Pablo Neruda*, page 131, by Pablo Neruda, translated by Margaret Sayers Peden, © 1990 by the Fundacion Pablo Neruda, published by the University of California Press; "Food Glorious Food," page 11, from the Columbia Pictures–Romulus Film *Oliver!* words and Music by Lionel Bart © copyright 1960 (renewed) Lakeview Music Co. Ltd., London, England, TRO—Hollis Music, Inc., New York, NY controls all publication rights for the U.S.A. and Canada, used by permission

Design by Forty-five Degree Design LLC

The information contained in this book is not intended to serve as a replacement for professional medical advice. Any use of the information in this book is at the reader's discretion. The author and the publisher specifically disclaim any and all liability arising directly or indirectly from the use or application of any information contained in this book. A health care professional should be consulted regarding your specific situation.

Designations used by companies to distinguish their products are often claimed as trademarks. In all instances where John Wiley & Sons, Inc., is aware of a claim, the product names appear in Initial Capital or ALL CAPITAL letters. Readers, however, should contact the appropriate companies for more complete information regarding trademarks and registration.

For general information about our other products and services, please contact our Customer Care Department within the United States at (800) 762-2974, outside the United States at (317) 572-3993 or fax (317) 572-4002.

Wiley also publishes its books in a variety of electronic formats. Some content that appears in print may not be available in electronic books. For more information about Wiley products, visit our web site at www.wiley.com.

Library of Congress Cataloging-in-Publication Data:
Miller, Sloane.
    Allergic girl : adventures in living well with food allergies/Sloane Miller.
      p. cm.
    Includes bibliographical references and index.
    ISBN 978-0-470-63000-6 (cloth);   ISBN 978-0-470-93084-7 (ebk.);
    ISBN 978-0-470-93085-4 (ebk.);   ISBN 978-0-470-93098-4 (ebk.)
      1. Food allergy—Popular works. I. Title.
  RC596.M55   2011
  616.97'5—dc22

                                                  2010046366

Printed in the United States of America
10 9 8 7 6 5 4 3 2 1

contents

foreword

by Julia E. Bradsher, PhD, MBA

Over the past ten years, as I have worked in the world of food allergies and anaphylaxis, I have encountered thousands of people who are living with and managing their own or their child's food allergies. Some of those I have met are truly living life to the fullest both in spite of and because of their food allergies. Sloane Miller, aka Allergic Girl, is one of those people. Sloane brings to this book expertise as an adult living with potentially life-threatening food allergies; as a social worker who works with adults, children, and families trying to manage their food allergies; as a true connoisseur of eating out in Manhattan; and, finally, as a gifted communicator. Wrapped around these areas of expertise, Sloane infuses this book with her joie de vivre.

As the CEO of FAAN, the Food Allergy and Anaphylaxis Network, I have the opportunity to speak to a large number of groups and audiences about food allergies and the importance of properly managing them in a number of settings. One of my favorite types of groups to speak to about food allergies are restaurant owners. I had the chance to be on a panel with Sloane about food allergies and eating out, at the International Restaurant and Foodservice Show of New York. During the panel, I was able to experience, firsthand, Sloane's zeal for making eating out not only accessible but truly a pleasurable experience for people with potentially life-threatening food allergies. In addition, Sloane also provides important insight and guidance on empowering and supporting yourself; navigating relationships with family, friends, and lovers; and being a part of the world in which you live. Whether you are an adult with a food allergy or a parent of an emerging adult, this book is a fantastic resource.

In addition, the book is fun and engaging to read. Sloane intersperses her insightful personal stories and the stories from others to illustrate the points she makes about managing and living with food allergies. She provides practical information in a style that makes you feel like you are sitting right there with her in a conversation.

There is an increase in the number of people with food allergies, and there is also a growing awareness of food allergies and their seriousness. For some, you are learning for the first time that your child has a potentially life-threatening food allergy. For others, you are an adult who has been living with food allergies your entire life, or you are an adult who has just learned that you have an adult onset food allergy. Regardless of your situation, Sloane Miller has written a book that is both practical and personal in providing you with insight, knowledge, and firsthand recommendations for how to navigate the world of food allergies. I hope you will use this book as a resource as you, too, live your life to the fullest.

Julia E. Bradsher, PhD, MBA, is the chief executive officer of FAAN, the Food Allergy and Anaphylaxis Network in Fairfax, VA.

a note to the reader

Many passages in this book are based on my memory. To the best of my ability, I confirmed these memories with outside sources. When there has been a consolidation of conversations, time or events, places or people's names, it was to protect the privacy of family, friends, and coaching clients. As for medical details, to the best of my knowledge they are accurate at the time of this writing. Consult with your personal physician and/or allergist as to the best course of action for you.

acknowledgments

My agent, Stéphanie Abou, has been the dearest friend, confidant, champion, hand holder, fashion consultant, and literary agent supreme since our first lunch back in 2004. Words cannot express my gratitude for her dedication to me and this project and my deep appreciation for her friendship. Editor and fellow allergic girl Christel Winkler saw the need for a book about the food-allergic community and snapped this up from the start. She is my inspiration to travel more and be an even better allergic girl. Thank you to the production, design, marketing, publicity, and sales teams at John Wiley & Sons for their hard work and endless enthusiasm in making this book a beautiful reality. Thank you to Lisa Burstiner, production editor extraordinaire, for shepherdessing me through the thorny copy-editing brambles.

Thank you to Fabrizio di Piazza, my strategic communications lead at DIP-INC, for believing in the mission of my work and helping me bring it to life. From his keen and thoughtful editorial eye to his attentive and forward-looking counsel, he has truly been a valued partner.

Thank you to legal expert and Lenox Girl Joyce Sydnee Dollinger, Esquire, who made the impossible maze of lyrics permissions possible.

Thank you to early readers Aimee Katz Zipkin, Dr. Arthur Spielman, Dr. Bonnie Jacobson, Dr. Carolyn Ellman, Marlene

Spielman, and Dr. Mathew Greenhawt, all of whom gave generously of their time to ensure I was on the right track.

Thank you to my allergy and nutrition colleagues who graciously contributed their expertise: Dr. Clifford Bassett; Marion Groetch, MS, RD, CDN; Marlisa Brown, MS, RD, CDE, CDN; and Dr. Matthew Greenhawt.

To my allergy, asthma, and food-allergy nonprofit colleagues, who make coping with food allergies a little easier, in particular: Mike Tringale at AAFA; Brian Oliver at Asthma and Allergy Friendly; Julia Bradsher, Jennifer Love Roeder, and the team at FAAN; Gwen Smith and the team at *Allergic Living* magazine; and Steve Rice and the team at FAI. Thank you for your support of both me and my work since the beginning.

Thank you to photographer and friend Kenneth Chen (kennethchenportraits.com) for the Allergic Girl blog and book cover photo. From that summer when I was your photography assistant until now, your eye has been a gift.

Thank you to photojournalist and friend David Handschuh (davidhandschuh.com) for a gorgeous author shot.

To my Allergic Girl blog readers, who, for the last five years, have let me know every day that we are all in this together. Without your readership and support there wouldn't have been a book: this is for you.

To my fellow bloggers, who welcomed me with open arms back in those early days, in particular: Alisa Fleming, Cybele Pascal, Erin Smith, Gina Clowes, Isaiah Benjamin, Janeen Zumerlin, Karina Allrich, Kelly Courson, and Shauna James Ahern. Thank you for all that you continue to do for all of us. To my many food-allergy blogger colleagues who have since joined the blogosphere and Twittersphere and helped to make the food allergy–free community feel a little less isolated and a lot more fun, thank you for all that you do every day.

To my private food-allergy coaching clients, consulting clients, and Worry-Free Dinners members who take that crucial leap to start trusting again and expanding your lives—working with you has expanded and enriched my life, thank you.

To the many restaurants and chefs nationally who have embraced my Worry-Free Dinners program and me personally: thank you for creating safe places for the food-allergic community to dine again and again.

I'm indebted to the many wonderful teachers I've had throughout my life who encouraged my love of learning: Oksana Solomczak, Abby Dubow, Nancy Blumenthal, Barbara Pulver, Jose Moreno-Lacalle, Steve Diner, Hugo Mahabir, Carl Barenboim, Karin Lesnik-Oberstein, Jason Shinder, Peggy Atkinson, Dr. Gerald Landsberg, and Dr. Jeffrey Seinfeld.

My parental Team Sloane offered unconditional love and support every step of the way: Harrice Simons Miller, Gary Jay Miller, Patty Madden Miller, Susie Simons Fasbinder, George Fasbinder, Dr. Bonnie Jacobson, Dr. Lenard Jacobson, Marlene Spielman, Dr. Arthur Spielman, Connie Emmerich, Nina Nathanson, Dr. Carolyn Ellman, and Jonathan Flaks.

My grandparents, Bernard Dine Simons, Beatrice Lillian Simons, Sidney Jay Miller, and Anne Kalmikoff Miller taught me to be expanding, always; they are all very much missed.

Loving friends offered support during the book-writing process in ways I couldn't have anticipated. Love and thanks to Ami Hoffman for daily xoxos; Christopher Hudson for his eternal "Yes, honey. Yes!"; Danielle Amedeo for harmonizing beautifully in song and in life; Josh Behar for being the best guy's guy a girl could want; Ta-Tanisha James for noticing that I've been working out my upper arms (and noticing everything else); and Yael Sonia Pomper for hosting our Lenox Girl brunches, always allergen-free.

And finally, thank you to my lifelong loves: Aimee Katz Zipkin, Tami di Piazza, Steve E. Smith, Isabel Rose, Kern J. Eccles, and Stéphanie Abou Cantor, who are on every page of this book and in every page of my life.

prologue

Yes, I am braver than I was. You asked me if I had
changed; I have changed in that way.

—Catherine Sloper, *Washington Square* by Henry James

"Do you feel that? Is my face . . . bumpy?"

"Mmm, I dunno," LT said as he nuzzled my neck.
"But it feels . . . itchy."

LT wasn't paying much attention. How could I blame him?
I adore kissing, too. It's like the best conversation you've ever had,
and with the right partner I just want to "talk" all night.

That evening, LT was at my house for dinner. We had dined
and were lounging, feeling relaxed and content. It was the perfect
time for a kiss, or a few hundred. Deep, tongue kisses. Soft pecks.
Exposed skin was fair game for affection. The date was heating up,
and my skin was tingling all over from excitement. Or was that
itching?

1

At first, I dismissed my unbelievably itchy face and neck as a fleeting reaction to beard stubble. However, what had been a slight tickle quickly progressed to a throbbing wave of itchy insistence— adamant, unrelenting, and getting worse.

I brought LT into the bathroom, and we looked in the mirror together. In the bright light of the tiled room, I was shocked to discover that I was covered in hives. Big welts and small pinpoints; my mouth was a Vandyke of red. My cheeks, both sides of my neck, my clavicle, and my right shoulder—everywhere LT had kissed me—was covered. I was also wheezing. Forget about looking hot; I looked like a smallpox victim. I was stunned.

It had been three years since I'd gotten hives from kissing someone. The last time, the rash from the salmon-tinged saliva trail had gone away on its own, quickly, and there had been no wheezing.

Not this time. Now there was no time for feeling embarrassed. I had to figure out what was going on and make it stop.

I have food allergies. I'm allergic to tree nuts and salmon.

Earlier that evening, I had casually informed LT about what to do in case of a food-allergic reaction. I showed him where my medications were kept, showed him the autoinjector of epinephrine and how to administer it, and mentioned that Benadryl is the first thing I should take if I was feeling allergic.

Because I was feeling extra relaxed, I revealed to LT the allergic signs that only someone who knows me extremely well would recognize. "I may not realize that I'm having an allergic reaction," I said. "I may just start itching. Or red hives may show up that you'll see before I do. I may start clearing my throat or may start complaining of itchy ears. If you see or hear any of that happening, tell me to take Benadryl." How prophetic.

Now, in the bathroom, I gazed dumbstruck at my red and bumpy self. LT, who was putting cold compresses on my neck, had been saying, "Take your antihistamine." I ignored him, intensely focused on my face and neck and not on the increasing symptoms. He finally insisted, "Please take the Benadryl, you're starting to freak me out." Thank goodness he had paid attention.

I took the little pink pill and used my rescue inhaler. While we waited for the effects to kick in, we talked through the possible causes. What had he put on his face that day? Dove soap and Neutrogena—no problems there. We ate dinner together—take-out food from a restaurant that I know and trust. His dish contained neither nuts nor fish. The server, knowing my allergies, specifically told me that LT's dish was safe for me, too. Then we ran through what LT had eaten earlier that day.

Cashews.

Only a few, in a trail mix and hours earlier. Since then, LT had eaten a cashew-free meal, which, according to current research, is the best way to rid one's mouth of a potential allergen. But this reaction wasn't because of proteins in his saliva; there was cashew residue in his beard.

Thirty minutes after I took the antihistamine and used the rescue inhaler, took a cool shower, and applied some topical cortisone cream, the bumps started to smooth out and the wheezing subsided. LT stayed the night to make sure things didn't flare up, and, well, we *were* still on a date. However, it wasn't exactly the kind of date either of us had had in mind.

the food-allergic community

Thirty years ago, severe food allergies were a rare diagnosis. Now, according to the Food Allergy and Anaphylaxis Network (FAAN), the accepted number is that twelve million of us are diagnosed with food allergies, which is one in every twenty-five Americans. (FAAN extrapolated this number from a combination of data from the Centers for Disease Control and Prevention and the National

Institute of Allergy and Infectious Diseases, then applied those studies to U.S. Census Bureau data.)

More and more Americans are going to their doctors and allergists with complaints of adverse reactions to food or suspected food-allergy concerns and receiving a diagnosis of food allergy. (A May 2010 *New York Times* article stated that up to thirty million Americans believe they have food allergies.)

The American Academy of Allergy, Asthma and Immunology (AAAAI) states on its Web site that the most common food-allergic reactions can include hives, a rash, or red itchy skin; a stuffy or itchy nose; sneezing; itchy and teary eyes; and respiratory distress. Other reactions can include vomiting, stomach cramps or diarrhea, and angioedema, or swelling. The most severe allergic reaction, however, is anaphylaxis (shock), the signs of which can include throat tightness, wheezing, trouble breathing or swallowing, hives or swelling, vomiting or diarrhea, a dip in blood pressure or loss of consiousness, and possibly death.

Ninety percent of food-allergic reactions are the direct result of ingesting foods common in the American diet: eggs, milk, wheat, peanuts, tree nuts, soy, fish, and shellfish. For millions, ingesting even a speck of any of these foods can mean a mild to severe immunological reaction. The U.S. Food and Drug Administration (FDA) states that there are 125,000 hospitalizations annually due to food allergies, and 14,000 of these are due to anaphylaxis.

According to a study published in the *Journal of Allergy and Clinical Immunology*, two hundred Americans die annually from food allergies, but this number is considered by the medical community to be the result of gross underreporting.

To avoid severe allergic reactions, millions of adults opt out of life's pleasures: kissing, dinner dates, social engagements, holidays and other celebrations, business lunches, and traveling to far-flung destinations—in other words, anywhere that food is involved, and that's pretty much everywhere. Even when they opt in, food-allergic adults are often actively fearful, anxious, or nervous. They can also feel ashamed, embarrassed, marginalized, isolated, lonely, and different because of their dietary restrictions. They often suffer in silence.

the allergic girl

That was me until a few years ago. I was born allergic, and a certain part of me simply accepted that this was my lot. When I was a child, I didn't advertise my food allergies to friends, extended family, schoolmates, or, when I was older, dates and boyfriends; it was a secret shame. With food allergies, environmental allergies, and allergic asthma, my body betrayed me at every turn. I'd invariably get sick from the food, the dust, or someone's dog. I rarely disclosed that I was ill. I did my best to handle it on my own; however, I was an allergic time bomb. It was never a question of *if* but always of *when*.

The worst part of having allergies was, and still is, being blamed for it. The prevailing feeling among casual acquaintances and even extended family has been that I was responsible for being allergic, that I could somehow control my allergic reactions, that I was faking the severity of an allergic response, or, worst of all, that I just wanted the attention.

There is no fakery here. I'd love to be able to eat anything I want at any time; however, that's just not how it is. The kind of attention that food allergies elicit is not the positive kind. It's a white-hot spotlight on a vulnerability. It's all eyes on you. No one wants that kind of attention. No one wants to be allergic to food.

So how did I go from being a shy, ashamed allergic girl, whose closest childhood friends often didn't know she had food allergies, to the Allergic Girl in the above story, who told her date how to take care of her in an emergency, who had an allergic reaction that did not prevent a romantic sleepover, and who then got a thank-you call from the guy the next day? (It's a feat, I know.) This is the journey of this book.

please don't pass the nuts

I started a blog called Please Don't Pass the Nuts in August 2006 to find others like me who are dealing and coping with food allergies and food intolerances. A licensed social worker since 2000, I opened a private food-allergy coaching, consulting, and advocacy practice, Allergic Girl Resources, Inc., in 2007. Then, in 2008, I launched my membership-based food-allergy dining club, Worry-Free Dinners. The blog, the private consulting and coaching practice, the dining club, and this book all serve one goal: to assist the food-allergic community members to live their best lives.

I hear one question over and over: How does a food-allergic person live a full life dictated by what he or she can't eat? My goal in writing this book is to tell you the basics of exactly *how* I do it and, most important, how *you* can, too. My premise is simple and actionable: Once you take your needs seriously, others will, too. Said another way, once you realize that you are entitled to your feelings, that your health is paramount and your medical needs are valid, those around you will support you.

The actions based on my premise are as follows:

1. Connect to your food-allergy needs without shame, embarrassment, or apology.
2. Communicate those needs clearly, assertively, and graciously.
3. Recognize that you have options and that there is always a way to get what you need.

I have organized this book into three parts. The first part is about you, your medical diagnosis, creating a positive doctor-patient relationship, and connecting to your feelings about your diagnosis. The second part is about the four most important relationships in your life: family, friends, lovers, and food. The third part combines your self-awareness, your support systems, and your new relationships and launches you into real-world scenarios scripted from my life and the lives of my generous food-allergy coaching clients and blog readers.

The concepts and strategies contained in this book are meant to grow with you. They are big and bold and may be unfamiliar or even daunting. Take these strategies step-by-step. Reread a sentence or a section. Try something out a few times, make it your own—as the recording artist Missy Elliott says, "Flip it and reverse it"—and then go to the next step or suggestion.

go boldly into your new life

I'm a practice-what-I-preach mental health–care worker, writer, advocate, and blogger. I dine out, I attend family events, I travel, and I date—all while having food allergies. Because I utilize the tools of education, self-awareness, and a support system, my experiences are successful and enjoyable. This is the result of a lifetime of hard work to get to a happier, healthier, expanding place. My suggestion is to start where you are now. Let the book sink in. Claim your food-allergic past and get ready to move on to your bright food-allergic future.

part one

you

1

the
allergic girl

I love food. I mean, I *really* love food. I love picking out a perfectly ripe avocado, its subtle green flesh creamy and glorious. I love roasted asparagus in the spring with olive oil, salt, fresh lemon zest, and lemon juice. Still-warm mozzarella from my local cheesemonger. Braised short rib, the meat fork-tender. Baked Rome apples à la mode. Onions and mushrooms frying in butter. Lamb chops. Toasted (okay, burned) marshmallows. Root beer floats. I could go on.

Some of my happiest and most satisfying, comforting, and sexiest memories have centered around the buying, making, and consuming of food.

But some of my scariest and most life-threatening, traumatizing, frustrating, and infuriating moments have also centered around the buying, making, and consuming of food.

I hate food. The prospect of going to a new restaurant sends me into a little panic. What will I be able to eat? What if I can't find anything? What if the server gives me the eye roll when I tell him or her about my allergies?

I dread going to dinner parties when I don't know the host or the menu. I'll simply have a bite before I go as insurance, but it's still kind of a drag.

What if my date just ate sushi and leans in for a big wet kiss? Do I lean back and say, "I don't think so"? Oh, *that's* a huge turn-on.

I despise not being able to pop anything I want into my mouth without thinking about it.

Holidays involve too much work. I know Aunt Bea meant well, but no, I can't pick the nuts off the Jell-O mold, and no, using the same now-nutty spoon from that Jell-O mold to serve me some mashed potatoes doesn't work. I'll pass, thanks.

Love, hate, dread, joy—my relationship to food is complex, colored by both trauma and pleasure. You too? I thought so.

flying blind

Most of the food-allergic reactions that emerged after toddlerhood (like salmon, eggplant, and melon) took me by complete surprise. I continued to eat the foods to which I was allergic, thinking small, kidlike thoughts such as "This must just be me," or "I'm eating this in the wrong way," or "This is how you're supposed to feel when you eat that food: your throat itches, your ears itch, and you can't swallow," or "This is all just *normal*, right?" I was in a sea of alone, an only child with lots of thoughts and internal explanations for what was happening. Many times I didn't tell anyone I was having a reaction—I didn't know it was an allergy.

On a basic level, I had no idea how food allergies worked. None. This wasn't something that was taught in school. I don't remember a doctor telling my parents or me much, except to keep me away from tree nuts. There was no Internet, and it never occurred to anyone to look up food allergies in the library—not that there were any kids' books about food allergies. I knew I had to stay away from tree nuts, and that was it. No one explained what to watch out for, what a food allergy is, how it affects you, or what to do in an emergency. There were no national consumer-support organizations. Autoinjectors of epinephrine weren't marketed until I was in middle school, and even then no one prescribed them to me. It wasn't medical negligence; it simply wasn't medical protocol.

Ironically, by the time I was diagnosed with allergic asthma at age four, I was well educated by my doctor and my parents. I used that education, common sense, and firsthand experience shrewdly. It told me what to avoid, when an attack was coming on, and what to do in an emergency. But food allergies? Beyond *maybe* taking an antihistamine, there was little education, guidance, or assistance. When it came to food allergies, I was flying blind. Everything I ate was a potential allergen, and more times than not, as a child, I was allergic.

online support

There are now excellent and reliable consumer-friendly resources available online for food allergies. Use them through your food-allergic journey to find board-certified allergists, medical information, chef cards, emergency plans, and much more.

- American Academy of Allergy Asthma and Immunology (AAAAI.org)
- American College of Allergy, Asthma, and Immunology (ACAAI.org)
- Anaphylaxis Canada (Anaphylaxis.ca)
- Asthma and Allergy Foundation of America (AAFA.org)
- Food Allergy Anaphylaxis Network (Foodallergy.org)
- Food Allergy Initiative (FAIUSA.org)

my allergic history

The family story is that when I was switched from breast milk to cow's milk, I developed a rash on my cheeks. My pediatrician, Dr. W., recognized this as a milk allergy, and I was switched to a soy formula. (The milk allergy disappeared by the time I was a toddler.) The FDA says that 90 percent of food-allergic reactions happen in response to eight common foods: eggs, dairy, wheat, peanuts, tree nuts, fish, shellfish, and soy. According to allergists, however, a person can be allergic to anything at any time.

My next allergic reaction, which I remember distinctly, was when I was two years old. I was at my Bubby's (grandmother's) house on Long Island, and there was an open jar of mixed nuts on the kitchen counter. I zoomed into the kitchen, grabbed a handful of nuts, popped them into my mouth, and zoomed out. When I ran back into the kitchen a few minutes later to grab some more, my Bubby was there, waiting. She looked at my face, and her eyes popped out of her head like a cartoon character. My lips and face had blown up. Immediately, she rushed me to the pediatrician in town, who gave me liquid cortisone, diagnosed me as allergic to tree nuts, and said, "Stay away."

That was the sole prescription and the only information we had for years.

food allergy defined

According to Dr. Matthew Greenhawt, MD, of the Division of Allergy and Clinical Immunology at the University of Michigan Medical School, "A food allergy is a clinical disorder based on clearly defined, repeatable symptoms that are directly attributable to a specific food ingestion. These symptoms must occur within a specific time period related to ingestion or contact with a particular food. The most important part of making such a determination is the clinical history—what actually happened or happens when a particular person ingests or comes in contact with a particular food."

a cheater's tale

I did try a tree nut again—once, and on purpose. I was eight years old. It was at a family dinner in an Italian restaurant in New York City's Little Italy, and I ordered tartufo for dessert. I remember asking if it had nuts, and the server said, "Filberts" (hazelnuts). I ordered it, anyway, out of earshot of my mother. I wanted to try it, to see if I was still allergic to nuts. Tartufo is two or three flavors of ice cream, and there can be fruit or nuts in the center. It's often enrobed in chocolate. Mine arrived, and I bit into the ice cream and some of the filbert. I had only the tiniest amount.

What happened next was a blur. There was a frenzied dash through Chinatown to find an open pharmacy that carried an antihistamine. We ended up at the local emergency room, and I was wheezing. I was given a shot of epinephrine, and then I sat on a hospital bed, white as a sheet and shaking, while I was observed. The wheezing subsided and I was out of danger, but I had learned my lesson. I was still allergic to tree nuts, no cheating allowed.

fish, vegetables, and fruits

I discovered, through ingestion and very distinct reactions, that I was allergic to fish (salmon, in particular), melon (cantaloupe and honeydew), and eggplant. When I was sixteen, during a medical intake with an allergist, Dr. M., I casually mentioned that I was having an odd reaction when I ate salmon. Dr. M. did a prick test and said the fateful words that I'm sure many of you have heard about your allergic reactions: "You are the most allergic person I've ever seen to salmon. Promise me you'll stay away from it." I've had no problem keeping that promise.

Eggplant gives me the same funny throat feeling, itchy and allergic. I found that out while eating vegetable couscous at a restaurant when I was a preteen. Many of the nightshade veggies

oral allergy syndrome

According to the American Academy of Allergy, Asthma, and Immunology: "Oral allergy syndrome (OAS) is a reaction to certain raw or fresh fruits or other foods that occurs in people who have been sensitized to airborne pollen. The syndrome is caused by a cross reactivity between airborne pollen proteins (tree, grass, weeds, plants) and proteins in fruits or vegetables. In people who are already allergic to pollen, the body's immune system sees a similarity between the proteins of pollen and those of the food, and triggers a reaction."

(tomatoes, potatoes, eggplants, and bell peppers) don't sit well with me. Eating a ripe tomato can give me what I call *funky mouth*: it feels as though I've eaten a razor blade. Bell peppers can give me a funny feeling on my palate, but with potatoes I'm fine. Some of the fruits with pits (like peaches, nectarines, and plums) give me that itchy-mouth feeling, especially when they are ripe; tropical fruits, such as mangoes and pineapples, do the same. Cooking the fruits can help, but sometimes it doesn't. My issues with pit fruits may be related to the time of year they are consumed; this is called oral allergy syndrome.

allergy testing

When I was two and diagnosed as allergic to nuts, there were no reliable blood tests available. Skin tests (either a scratch or a prick test) were available, but I was and still am very topically sensitive. My pediatric allergist, Dr. F., focused his education and treatment suggestions on my then moderate asthma; food allergies weren't a strong focus. He suggested a food challenge in his office that I declined. It was too scary, especially after the filbert incident.

At sixteen, I switched from pediatrics to an adult allergist's office. Dr. M. did a series of scratch tests based on my allergic history. I reacted immediately and severely to all of the allergens he tested. It took three days to recover: three days of huge welts, antihistamines, and the use of my inhaler. The tests confirmed all of my childhood allergies as intact and intense. He did not suggest a food challenge.

Testing alone never tells the full food-allergic picture, however. An allergist told me an illuminating story. He blood-tested himself for ragweed and was shown to have the highest response possible to that common allergen. However, he had *never* experienced an allergic reaction to ragweed. You can test positive for an allergen and yet never experience a reaction. Allergy testing can give you a sense of an allergic possibility, but it's nothing definite. When I did the scratch tests with Dr. M., they were based on my allergic history and confirmed what I already knew: I was highly allergic. The bottom line is that no single test, other than a direct food challenge (eating a suspected allergen under direct medical supervision), can diagnose someone as food allergic.

From elementary school to high school, I uncovered more food allergies through ingesting new foods. Subsequently, there were more foods to avoid and more coping skills required to get through a day: negotiate a sleepover or figure out how to stay safe on a school trip or during sleepaway camp. I became an expert Allergic Girl on how to avoid my allergy triggers whenever possible, how to explain my allergic needs to others, how to cook safe foods for myself, and how to advocate to those around me.

panic is no picnic

As I aged and developed strategies to cope, I also developed a juicy case of generalized anxiety. It's natural to feel panicky after a severe allergic reaction. It's also natural to be concerned about when the next one might crop up. Danger lurks in an unlabeled walnut brownie at the school dance or in a nutty mole sauce at the Mexican restaurant. In my adolescence, I was panicky about an anticipated allergic reaction *and* an actual allergic reaction. Sometimes they were one and the same and thus very difficult to distinguish.

Feelings of panic only exacerbated the food-allergic symptoms, masked them, or created symptoms that might not have been there (see chapter 3). With a lot of personal work, dietary vigilance, a great support system, and the strategies I will delineate later, I am able to manage the anxiety and do everything I want to do.

allergies now

When I was growing up, I was the only food-allergic kid I knew. There were no 504 plans that allow a child with a severe food allergy to be protected under the Individuals with Disabilities Education Act (IDEA) by requesting a nut-free environment at school, for example. I carried my inhaler in the pocket of my school uniform. There were no autoinjectors of epinephrine for me at the nurse's station or anywhere else. If I had any reactions at school or on a playdate, I was the one who was responsible for taking care of it.

My teachers, though sweet, wouldn't have known what to do; there was no food-allergic safety training. There were no cell phones for reaching parents in an emergency, just services or secretaries with whom to leave messages. It's undeniable that things have changed radically in a generation.

The question remains: Why are there so many allergies worldwide, and why now? The answer is murky even within the food-allergic medical community. As of this writing, there's no consensus. As an allergist colleague said to me recently: "It's real, it's documented, and it's happening. We just don't know why."

Dr. Matthew Greenhawt MD, of the Division of Allergy and Clinical Immunology at the University of Michigan Medical School, supplied me with six current possible theories about why there are so many food allergies diagnosed now:

- *Awareness.* Part of the rise in the rate is due to better awareness of the issue, which has increased the number of individuals tested and diagnosed.
- *Better hygiene.* With less infectious disease, the body may be shifting away from cytokines (immune factors) that fight infection to cytokines that promote allergy formation. Evidence for this theory is seen in sub-Saharan Africa, where there are high rates of infectious disease but low rates of allergy and asthma. In Westernized countries, the opposite is seen.
- *Pollution.* Smog and diesel exhaust are known to promote allergy-forming cytokines among chronically exposed children. This may contribute to the rise in rates among inner-city populations, for whom exposure to such particles is greater than for those who live in suburban or rural areas.
- *Food processing.* Technological advances in food preparation may be increasing the expression of certain food allergens.
- *Timing of introduction of food.* There is great debate about whether babies should eat high-risk allergens in their first year or wait until they are older. The introduction of such foods in the first year of life may be associated with lower rates of allergy, although there is no clear consensus.
- *Genetics.* Given that allergies and asthma do tend to run in certain families, there may be a gene or a set of genes that contributes to this. There may also be genes that suppress allergy and asthma. One's environment may influence what genes are expressed, further confounding this theory. For now, however, there is simply no firm answer to why there is a food-allergy epidemic.

treatment options: buyer beware

So here we are. Millions of us have adverse reactions to common foods. What's the treatment? The best and only treatment available right now is *avoidance*. That's it. Once you're educated on how to do it, it's free. However, with the increase in diagnosis and the inevitable increase in major media attention, there's been a marked increase in hucksters offering promises of saving you from certain food-allergy discomfort or disaster. More and more snake-oil salespeople are waiting to prey upon the food-allergic community's deepest fears and grandest hopes. Like good rainmakers, they say what anyone would want to hear: "I have the cure, treatment, or answer." The old adage is true here: If it sounds too good to be true, it probably is. Resist the temptation to believe, buy, invest, try, sample, or in any way participate in food-allergy treatment scams.

Remember, as of right now there is no cure for food allergies.

food-allergy research

If you're interested in learning more about the current food-allergy research, or even being part of a human trial, the following hospitals are part of Consortium of Food Allergy Research (CoFAR), cosponsored by the National Institutes of Health (NIH) and the National Institute of Allergy and Infectious Diseases (NIAID):

Duke University Medical Center
Johns Hopkins University
Mount Sinai Medical Center, Jaffe Food Allergy Institute
National Jewish Health
University of Arkansas for Medical Sciences

For further information on CoFAR, contact the Statistical and Clinical Coordinating Center at (301) 251-1161 or at cofar@emmes.com.

You may have heard of some "cures" on the horizon from the medical community or through national media outlets. These cures are in fact therapies or treatments to lessen the severity of a potential reaction. The trials look promising, but as of right now, no treatment can eliminate food allergies.

Your best tools for staying healthy and reaction-free in the present are education, common sense, body awareness, emergency medications, and plans for multiple life scenarios. Education comes in many forms, including reliable medical information and an excellent allergist. Not all doctors are created equally, though. Finding the right doctor—and, in this case, allergist—is a process that is well worth undergoing.

allergic girl's food-allergy basics

- A food allergy is the immune system's response to a food that the body perceives as foreign and dangerous.
- The FDA identifies eight common foods that cause 90 percent of food-allergic reactions, but someone can be allergic to virtually anything.
- Typical food-allergy symptoms are itching, hives, swelling skin, flushing, wheezing, coughing, swelling of lips or throat, vomiting, diarrhea, a decrease in blood pressure, shock, and throat closure. In very rare cases, these can lead to death.
- It is vital that you never downplay, ignore, dismiss, or disregard a food-allergic symptom, reaction, or response.
- There is no clear consensus on why there are so many allergies now, but it is real and it is documented.
- Effective food-allergy treatments are being researched, but currently there is no food-allergy cure.
- The most effective food-allergy treatment is strict avoidance of the allergens.

2

team you

I'm going to take your blood pressure, so try to relax
and not think about what a high reading might mean
for your chances of living a long, healthy life.

—David Sipress, cartoon "Blood Pressure,"
New Yorker, January 4, 2010

Click clack, click clack were the sounds of my mother's heels on the tile floor as we rushed to the office of Dr. W., my pediatrician. The office was down an interminable hallway, to a first-floor converted apartment in Peter Cooper Village in Manhattan. I hated going to the doctor's office, and my mother practically had to drag me down that hallway.

Dr. W. was the first to recognize that I was an allergic girl. My mother says that when I was an infant and developed a rash on my cheek, he immediately recognized it as a milk allergy, and I was switched to soy milk formula.

The apartment's former living room, now a waiting room, was perennially in shadow even though it faced the renowned Peter Cooper gardens. Your eyes needed to adjust quickly, or *snap*, you'd step on the toys strewn about on the floor. Two plastic, color-rubbed-off-in-all-of-the-worn-places rocking horses were suspended on large metal coils that creaked and whined; headless dolls in various states of disrepair and loved-up use, plastic parts of toys of yesteryear, and half-torn books were the detritus of this well-used, well-worn, pediatric doctor's waiting room.

Also in the big former living room was the desk of nurse A. She was Dr. W.'s foil. Whereas he was a gruff, no-nonsense doctor, she was a sweet and gentle nurse. He was tall and slim and wore tweeds (no lab coats) and wire-rimmed glasses; she was petite and curvy and wore a starched white uniform, her brown hair in a stiff blow-and-set. Some people just go together, and Dr. W. and Nurse A. just went together.

Dr. W. was intimidating. When I went into his office, he looked me straight in the eye and asked me how I was and what was wrong. Not many adults did that; I would discover later that not many pediatricians did that, either. My mother remembers fondly that Dr. W. seemed to forget her name, but he always remembered every detail about my health history and health care. I recall that even made a house call once when I was very little and very ill. He was conservative with medication and relied on time-tested practices; he wasn't experimental. Even though his demeanor seemed stern to me, every visit ended with a small plastic toy, the flash of a wry smile, and a very firm cheek pinch. Every single visit, without fail.

In hindsight, Dr. W. was the model of an excellent old-school pediatrician: calm, conservative, and trustworthy. His office consisted of one doctor: him. He had one nurse who managed the office, the patients, the payments, and the incessantly ringing phone. Dr. W. retired from fifty years of medical practice when I was ten years old, so we were forced to find a new pediatrician.

Little did I know what a precious commodity doctors like Dr. W. were and still are.

nameless in a group

From ten years old until I left for college at seventeen, I was with a pediatric group at the nearby teaching hospital. I did not have the luxury of a regular doctor. When I came in for appointments, I was given to whatever doctor was available. The office space was clinical and impersonal. There were definitely no presents at the end of visits and no pinches on the cheek. I often saw Dr. B., a soft-spoken person and an asthma specialist. He usually spoke directly to my mother, asking her about my symptoms or my care; he rarely addressed me directly.

uncle doctor

When I came home from college, I needed an internist. I didn't want a repeat of the experience of a large impersonal group of rotating doctors and office staff. I wanted a doctor who would know me the way Dr. W. did. I also wanted a doctor who would listen to me without judgment, who would be trustworthy and old-school. I wanted a doctor who wouldn't put me on hold with Muzak or, worse, a phone messaging system.

Through a doctor friend of the family, a pulmonologist's name was proffered: Dr. S. The first time I walked into the ground floor of his Upper East Side brownstone, a kindly bearded man gave me a jaunty hello. (Was that the doctor?) The office was homey and not clinical. There were plenty of magazines to flip through, and sunlight streamed in the bay windows. The friendly man was wearing khaki pants and hovered over the nurse's station. He and the nurse, in the white lab coat, were engaged in friendly banter. Clearly they liked working together; they were at ease around each other, and there was no tension in the office. I overheard the man in the khakis (yes, that was the doctor) ask who the next patient was.

I said, "I'm a friend of Dr. J.'s, and I think I'm next."

Dr. S. said, "Ah, but of course," in a silly accent and then "Okay, see you in a bit" as he zipped into the back rooms.

I could tell immediately that this doctor liked being in his office. He was a generally happy guy who was slightly informal yet still professional. Bonus: He had a personality. Extra bonus: His office consisted of just him and one nurse–office manager who handled everything. That was ringing some deep doctor bells I didn't even realize I had.

That first visit was in 1994. Dr. S. has been my primary-care physician ever since. Whether I call to ask a quick medical question or for an emergency, he picks up the line with a reassuring "Hello-o-o-o, Sloane! What's up?" During my annual exam, we usually chitchat (how's the family, how's work, did you have a nice holiday, did you read this new book?) before I go over my list of questions, issues, and concerns; it makes for a much more pleasant appointment. He has seen me through bouts of bronchitis and bouts of anxiety; I've seen him at synagogue and bumped into him on Broadway. He's like an uncle who happens to be my doctor. This has been a long-term and successful medical partnership for Team Sloane.

team you defined

What is Team Sloane? For that matter, what is a Team You? Team You is a network of supportive individuals who assist you in getting to the next happy step in your life. Reading this book qualifies; ergo, I am now part of Team You. Your family can be part of Team You. Loyal and loving friends are definitely part of Team You. Your romantic partner is a member of Team You. Your fantastic boss and your excellent coworkers can be part of your team. Your drinking buddies, your poker buddies, your book club, your racquetball club, your Sunday brunch girls, your Saturday basket-ball boys—they can all be part of Team You.

A crucial aspect of Team You, and the one that we are going to focus on right now, is your medical Team You. For those of us with food allergies, creating and maintaining a crack medical Team You is simply the best way to coordinate care. Whether you've had food allergies a long time and know what your allergies are or you suspect you have a food allergy and need a correct food-allergy diagnosis, everyone can use some help finding a great allergist to round out Team You.

The American Academy of Allergy, Asthma, and Immunology suggests on its Web site seeing an allergist for the following rea-sons: "If you think you are having an allergic reaction to food; for any allergic reaction that has an unclear cause; to confirm a suspected allergy; if you have limited your diet based on possible allergy to foods or additives; for advice on the best treatment and avoidance measures for food allergy; and for advice on ways to prevent potential food allergy."

I will add that you want an allergist with the most experience with food allergies as possible. You want an allergist who's upbeat and not all doom and gloom about a food-allergy diagnosis. You need an allergist who knows about reliable food-allergy testing

finding an allergist

You can find a qualified board-certified allergist through these reputable sources:

* American Academy of Allergy, Asthma, and Immunology: www.aaaai.org
* American College of Allergy, Asthma, and Immunology: www.acaai.org
* American Medical Association: www.ama-assn.org
* Your medical insurer or managed-care provider

and is able to execute those tests accurately. You need an allergist who can further educate you and your loved ones about food allergies and what to do in an emergency, who can create a plan of food-allergy action, and who will be available for questions or in an emergency.

the allergist works for you

It is a truth universally acknowledged: no one likes going to the doctor. As kids, we're dragged kicking and screaming into doctors' offices for the requisite pokes, prods, and shots, priming us not to like them. Very often, the moment we step over the threshold of any doctor's office, we're instantly time-warped into the childhood dimension: no power, no voice, no clue.

How do we stop shrinking into the floor when we enter the doctor's office? How do we stop becoming six years old all over again when our names are called to go into that little cold room? How do we take some control back over our health and our health care? As an adult, you have the power to choose the individual you want to help you get into (or stay in) the best health possible. Choose an allergist for Team You (or any medical health professional) by keeping some of the aspects described below in mind.

Doctors Are People, Too

Generally speaking, doctors have the drive to help and to heal complete strangers. They go through rigorous training and education to gain specialized knowledge, expertise, and experience, all to service that initial drive to help. (Also generally speaking, most doctors are scientists at heart.)

After all of that training, though, at the heart of it doctors are still people. They have biases, strengths, weaknesses, blind spots, annoying quirks, and tics. They can be sympathetic, funny, and creative; they can also be impatient, exhausted, and dismissive. Some doctors say the right thing to calm you down, give you the right medication in the right dosage, are excellent diagnosticians, know when to refer you to a specialist, and are super-duper people.

But not all doctors are compassionate or intelligent. Remember, they're human, not superhuman. Doctors are people first, with emotional baggage, family issues, societal pressures, and gaps in their medical knowledge. Most doctors, although perfectly lovely people, may not be bubbling over with personality. Some may not have great eye contact, and some may not have much capacity for small talk. This is not a reflection on a doctor's abilities, just on his or her social skills.

So along with understanding that doctors are people, too, it helps to recognize that the people who are drawn to the medical profession are not necessarily Mr. or Ms. Outgoing Social Butterfly. A retired well-known surgeon at a big New York City teaching hospital once told me, "The doctors with the biggest practices usually have better personalities but not better training." It's something to keep in mind.

The Ideal

As a Team You member, your doctor or allergist should listen to you and take note of your presenting problem; educate you about your disease, illness, or condition; and give you good advice and good specialist referrals. He or she should make time for you when you're sick, treat you with respect, listen to you about what you need and what your problems may be, and work in cooperation with you to help you find the right solution *for you*. You have the right to a doctor who listens to your needs and devises a plan you can understand and follow, whether you're being cared for in a community health center, a free walk-in clinic, a city-funded hospital, a managed-care physician's office, or a private doctor's office.

honesty is your main tool

The main role you play in Team You is to be honest with yourself about what kind of doctor you relate to best and then to talk with your medical team honestly about what you need. It sounds simple, but sometimes the simplest advice, like "Be honest," is the most difficult to implement. Part of being honest is knowing more about yourself and your feelings about doctors, health, and health care. Your job is to keep chipping away at it, be as honest as you can whenever you can, and then chip away some more.

Your ethnic background, your culture, your financial status, your family's views, your personal values, and your belief system all enter the mix when you're thinking about health, disease, treatments, cures, and medicine. Everyone is truly an individual, and the differences should be examined and respected.

Having a medical team is an ideal way to reach a goal of health; however, there are myriad ways to reach that goal. While honoring your belief systems, your values, your cultural heritage, and your background, consider your feelings, your objectives, and your ideals pertaining to health, disease, and medicine. It's worth thinking about some historical interactions with doctors and your family's overall impressions of the medical community as well.

Ask yourself some questions: Does your family believe in going to the doctor for a wellness visit? Does your family believe that you should visit the doctor only when you're sick and not beforehand? Would family members tease or even shame you now because you want to go a doctor for an evaluation? What would your family think if you said that the doctor is a member of a team that works for you?

Think it through; bring up some memories about the doctors of your past and how that is informing your feelings and behavior toward doctors now. You may be surprised to find that you have more memories or feelings about a doctor's visit than you thought.

Make a list, if you're moved to, either mentally or physically. Talk with a safe friend (see chapter 5 about how to create safe friends), a sibling, a cousin, or a parent about the doctor. Keep in mind where you have been, where you are now, and where you want to go in your relationship with medical professionals.

further questions to consider

Now that you've thought about who you are in that little examining room, let's talk more about the person sitting across from you. Who is this doctor, and who, in your ideal scenario, do you want him or her to be? (We may not achieve the ideal, but it's good to know what the ideal is.)

What qualities do you admire in your work colleagues, your boss, your parents, or your significant other? What kind of communication styles work well for you? Are you a tough-love gal? Are you a break-it-to-me-softly guy? Do you need lots of direct eye contact? Does too much eye contact make you uncomfortable? Do you need a doctor with a sense of humor? Would you rather see a doctor who is all tests and research? What about age, gender, and ethnic background? Do you want a seasoned professional, or do you prefer a newbie with all the latest tricks at his or her fingertips?

Do you prefer the kind of doctors you see on television, hear on the radio, read about on the Internet, or listen to on podcasts? Do you want a doctor with famous patients? Do you want a doctor who is actively doing research on your ailment? Do you care where your doctor went to undergraduate, graduate, or medical school? Do you prefer a doctor who wears a white lab coat and has books and degrees in his or her office? Do you like a doctor who wears street clothes, makes notes on a computer, uses social network media, is a big e-mailer, and gives you his or her cell phone number for emergencies? Whom do you want on your team? What sort of Team You teammate works best?

what kind of patient are you?

As the Caterpillar asked Alice in *Alice in Wonderland*, "Who are you?" Do you secretly hope that the doctor can just fix everything? Do you think that whatever the doctor says is mostly dictated by the pharmaceutical companies? Do you come in with reams of Internet research and challenge everything the doctor says? Do you find that you're struck mute the moment you step over the threshold and have to struggle to remember why you're even there?

There's no judgment here, just ask yourself: Who are you when you get into that room? Think it through; bring up some memories about the doctors of your past and how they inform your feelings and behavior toward doctors now. You may be surprised that you have more memories or feelings about a doctor's visit than you thought.

get some referrals

How do you find this new member of Team You? Word of mouth is one of the better ways to find an allergist, but just asking around won't get you the answer you need. When you ask friends for a recommendation, dig a little deeper. Ask some probing questions about why your friends like their doctors, not just "Are they 'good?'" *Good* is relative; what's good for one person ("She has the best magazines in the waiting room") may not be good for you. So go ahead, put on your Magnum P.I. mustache and get to the bottom of why this doctor is the one everyone loves.

Group e-mails for doctor referrals are easy to do and work well. Here's a sample e-mail:

Dear All,

I'm looking for a new allergist. Do you have one who you think is the best? If yes, can you tell me a little about why he or she is the best? For example: Does he return your calls promptly? Does she have a nice office staff? Is his office conveniently located? Does she have good professional referrals? Is he an excellent diagnostician? Can she pinpoint what the issue is and treat it? Does he have a kind bedside manner? Does she take your concerns seriously? Is he an active listener? Does she explain your diagnosis in language you can understand? Specific details would help me greatly. Thanks so much!

Best, Sloane

If you want to send out a social-network message, that can be equally effective. Gather the names of specialists and start doing some Internet searches. If a name comes up more than once, that might be an indicator that this is a doctor you would like.

interviewing doctors

Now that you have gathered a few names from different sources, it's time to interview these doctors. There are two ways to go: indirectly or directly. Read through all of the options presented below; on some days you might feel like just showing up and assessing, and on other days you'll be ready for a bolder approach. Both approaches are effective, and both will let you know whether this is the right team member for you.

Indirect Interviews

The easiest and least invasive sleuthing tool is an Internet search. Many doctor referral sites will ask for a fee, but often, if you dig a little deeper, you can find the right information without paying a fee. Here's what you're looking for: Where did the doctors go to medical school? Where did they do their internships and residencies? Are they board certified? (Don't go to any doctors who aren't.) Do they do research in your topic area? Have they written any articles you can access? Are there peer or patient reviews available? Does your medical insurer have online information about these doctors? Some insurers have started internal rating systems, so look for that information online as well.

The second indirect source is the doctor's office manager. These people have often been working at their offices for years and have fielded the kinds of questions you'll be asking. Ask to speak with the office manager directly (not the receptionist) about where the doctor trained, how many food allergy patients the doctor sees, office hours and after–office hours availability, any hospital affiliation, any recent publications, maybe even other patients you could talk to. If the office manager has none of this information, that could be telling; maybe the office has high turnover, or maybe it means nothing. The bottom line is that talking with the office manager can be less intimating than asking the doctor directly about these issues.

A third source of indirect but incredibly valuable information about any medical professionals—how they work and if that will work for you—is what their offices say about them. From your first Internet search to your first phone call, every step of the process will give you information about a doctor's practice. When dealing with new medical professionals, use all of your senses and your gut. Trust your intuition. "Spidey senses" aren't just for the cartoon character; you have them, too. They're excellent. Use them.

When you call for an appointment, be aware of the following: Does the office staff talk to you respectfully or hurriedly? Does the office keep you on hold longer than one minute? Does the staff seem efficient or confused? Do you get the sense that the staff is doing you a favor by giving you an appointment? Or do you sense that the staffperson answering the phone is patient and listening to your needs and doing his or her best to squeeze you in?

After you have made an appointment and arrive at the physical space, look around the office. Is it tidy, warm, and friendly? Is it cold, chaotic, disorganized, or grimy? Are the magazines in tatters, or are there at least three crisp copies of your favorite magazine waiting to be read? The front desk is the front line, an extension of the doctor. What is the staff like in person? Are the people friendly, warm, and caring? Is there a high turnover, or have the same people been there for years?

great doctor, less great office

Sometimes the office is not a reflection of the doctor's training, abilities, or personality. My allergist in high school, Dr. M., was a doctor's doctor and trained many of New York City's best allergists. He was an elegant man: his lab coat was bright white and pressed, his shoes were always shined, and his thick lustrous hair had not one strand out of place. His demeanor was calm and generally sunny, he talked to me directly and kindly, and he was a conservative clinician. I felt very good about his level of care.

His office, however, was one of the worst I have ever encountered. The wait to see him, even with an appointment, was typically four hours. I once waited six hours for my regular appointment; the staff was that disorganized. The cause seemed to be his office manager, who was also his wife. Whereas he was elegant, she was slovenly; whereas his hair was perfectly coiffed, hers made her look like a character from Jim Henson's *Fraggle Rock*; whereas he was all smiles, she was testy, grumpy, and wheezy.

The patient files, supposedly confidential, were spread everywhere in high, messy piles: on her desk, on her chair, and on the floor in a maze impossible to navigate. And she chain-smoked; a lit and ash-dropping cigarette dangled from her mouth at all times. The smoky office was certainly not conducive to happy lung health for we, the allergic and asthmatic patients. As much as I liked, respected, and trusted my allergist, I (and my lungs) couldn't tolerate the state of his office. After college, I looked elsewhere.

Who actually sees you? Are you being shunted off to a physician's assistant or, worse, to a partner whom you've never heard of rather than the doctor with whom you made the appointment? How many people do you have to go through to get to the actual doctor? Do you feel as though you've entered a Kafka novel: a labyrinth of white coats and no answers forthcoming?

Once you are brought into the little examining room and are face-to-face with the doctor, what do you feel: nervous, taken care of, intimidated, or at ease? Is the doctor prepared to talk to you? Does he speak to you in doctorese or in plain English? Does she answer your questions or simply tell you what she is going to do and leave the room? All this information will affect your relationship with this potential Team You member.

Direct Interviews

If you are ready for a bolder approach when looking for your best medical Team You member, I suggest interviewing the doctor. If you've never interviewed a doctor, I won't lie to you: it's not the most natural thing to do. Many of us feel intimidated or freeze up when talking to a doctor. It's understandable. They seem to have all of the answers to your problems in that manila folder of theirs. I have a coaching client whose blood pressure always shoots up when she sees her doctor. Another client forgets what the presenting issue is the moment he steps into that little white room. Again, it's very natural: doctors see this all the time.

Going to a doctor's office knowing that this person is a potential Team You member will help with the interview process. If you're wondering how a doctor will interpret being interviewed, the answer is that it depends. Some doctors might be offended; some doctors will take it in stride. Their reactions are just more information for you to consider about what kind of team member they would be. Try it; you can know only if you try. Ultimately, talking frankly with health-care professionals will give you the information you need to choose the right doctor for you.

What you ask your potential new Team You member depends on what your priorities are. Therefore, it's vital that you have a sense of what those needs are before you walk into the examining room. Go back to the section "Further Questions to Consider" and think through some of the answers or talk with a friend about what you really need in a doctor-patient relationship. Two important sample questions for a new doctor are the following: What is your experience pertaining to food allergies? How can I get in touch with you if I need you after office hours or on the weekends?

be honest with your doctor

Once you've selected a doctor, remember what I mentioned previously: your role in this partnership is to speak to your medical team with honesty, forthrightness, graciousness, and respect, with the full expectation of having those qualities reciprocated. A team works best when built upon a foundation of honesty. Your medical team can give you a proper diagnosis only if there is a real and honest assessment about what is going on with you.

On December 14, 2009, the *New York Times* confirmed the need for honesty in doctor-patient relations: "The importance of effective communication in that setting cannot be overemphasized. Accurate diagnosis and treatment of medical ailments depend on the doctor's clear understanding of the entire person who sits before her." Your medical partnership must start with honesty. Speak up about what you need, and more often than not your medical team will be able to help you in the right way.

If you feel uncomfortable, uncared for, unheard, or shunted off; if your calls are not returned, among other impolite transgressions: leave that office and take your business elsewhere. Yes, you read correctly. This is a business and you are the consumer. Equally important: this is your health. You are in control;

the doctor is there to help you. If you have been honest about your needs, if you have spoken directly and with courtesy to your doctor and his or her office staff and have not had that reciprocated, go elsewhere. It is worth the time and the effort to find the right person to join your team. More than worth it, it's vital to your continued good health.

talking to your doctor

Once you've made an appointment with your new doctor, it's best to come prepared. How do you even get a doctor to talk to you for ten minutes in this world of managed care? I asked Clifford W. Bassett, MD, FAAAAI, FACAAI, faculty, NYU School of Medicine and assistant clinical professor of medicine and otolaryngology, the Long Island College Hospital, SUNY Downstate Medical Center, New York, for his tips for making your visit efficient once you get into that little room with someone you like and trust.

* Have a summary of your past and recent medical symptoms and complaints written clearly, including a broad history of care, test results, and medication lists.
* Have some clear goals and objectives with regard to your active health issues.
* Understand the many benefits of a preventative approach to a variety of health and wellness issues.
* Have an updated list of current medications and supplements as well as names, addresses, and contact information of your active medical practitioners.
* Ask for recommendations to specialists who will explain and simplify the successful management of your specific health care concerns and illnesses.
* Have some knowledge about your insurance and pharmacy program formulary plans to know which are preferred medications before visiting the pharmacy.

diagnosis: head stuff

One of the first truly honest (and a little embarrassing) conversations I had with my primary case physician Dr. S. happened over the phone about two years after my first visit to his office. I called him at six o'clock in the morning, on a weekend, from a pay phone in Vermont. It was my first winter at graduate school. My chest had been tight for days, but that morning I woke up feeling as though someone were sitting on it. I wasn't wheezing, and I wasn't congested; I had no cough, no fever, no phlegm. I had brought my own bedding, and there were no animals in the dorms, so I probably wasn't allergic. I used my rescue inhaler, but it did nothing to alleviate the tightness. It felt like an emergency.

I called Dr. S.'s service, which connected me with the doctor. After he came on the line with a very sleepy "What's wrong, Sloane?", I described my symptoms (chest tightness), where I was (Bennington, Vermont; graduate school), and how long the symptoms had been going on (a few days). Dr. S. said, "I don't think it's asthma. I think it's head stuff."

Once I realized he was right—I wasn't wheezing but simply anxious and tense—I laughed with relief. I was able to relax, look at my situation calmly, and start having fun. A moment of embarrassment and vulnerability with my doctor cleared the path for the recognition of what was happening with my body and helped me to form other honest relationships with medical professionals. This short conversation positively reinforced that I would not be judged for my stark honesty, but I would be helped.

hi, i'm sloane, and i'm med phobic

Fast-forward to 2009, at the office of Dr. N., a pain-management specialist who utilizes both Western and Eastern techniques. After having years of honest conversations with Dr. S., I took another, even bolder step. I wrote on Dr. N.'s intake form, "No medication allergies known, but am med phobic." After going through a childhood filled with daily asthma and allergy medications, I really don't like taking medication if I don't have to or if there are alternatives. (However, I always take prescribed asthma or allergy medications.)

Writing "med phobic" on an intake form is personally revealing. It's also not something I'm particularly proud of, but I'm working on taking new medications and not worrying about improbable side effects or unlikely medication allergies. Writing "med phobic" on a form that stays in my medical file forever gave me an internal pang of vulnerability. I wondered whether this new doctor would judge me, or worse, think I was going to be a difficult patient and treat me differently (make that a double pang). All that judging was possible and even probable.

However, if I hadn't written "med phobic," if I hadn't been completely honest, and this pain-management doctor had prescribed pain medications and I didn't take them, I'd simply be a noncompliant patient. The doctor would not have been able to do a whole lot, in terms of my prescribed course of treatment. So even though I felt silly or even a little ashamed about this aspect of myself, I knew that this information would be vital for helping this doctor to help me.

The direct result of this level of honesty was that when discussing treatment options, the doctor offered two. One option was a painful series of steroid injections that have a 50 percent chance of eliminating pain and have serious side effects. The other was acupuncture, which is noninvasive, nonmedicinal, without side effects, and proven to be very effective for pain. I chose the latter, and because I had told my doctor that I was med phobic, he understood my decision without pressuring me.

Thus, a moment of vulnerability on my intake form smoothed the way for having a more open conversation about my pain treatment, rather than having a doctor who would recommend all kinds of medications I would never take. Bonus: Dr. N. told me

are you "med phobic"?

If you feel overly anxious, distressed, nervous, or avoidant about taking medications, I suggest you do the following:

- Talk through all of the treatment options with your medical provider.
- Talk through the possible versus the probable side effects with your medical provider.
- Use Internet searches about new medications judiciously—sometimes the information does more harm than good.
- If feasible, try the first dose in the doctor's office.
- Learn to recognize the signs of anxiety and panic versus the physiological side effects of medications. (See chapter 3 for more about anxiety.)
- If anxiety about a medication (new, old, rescue, or emergency) is interfering with normal life functioning, consider seeing a mental health professional for an evaluation.

that my honesty was helpful to him as a tool to better understand me and my needs. He even thanked me for that level of honesty.

allergic girl's prescription for team you

- Set out to create the best medical support team possible at this moment in time.
- Recognize that doctors are people, too. They have good days and bad days, strengths and weaknesses. Find a doctor who suits you best.
- Create insight into what kind of patient you are and what kind of doctor would be best for you.
- Do your homework to find a qualified medical professional. Assess your potential candidates and their offices for suitability.

- Be honest with yourself and with your doctor; it's the best way he or she can help you.
- Arrive at medical appointments prepared with questions, research, medical history, and current needs.
- The food-allergic patient needs a correct diagnosis, disease education, an emergency plan, medicine prescriptions, instructions on how and when to use the medications, and consistent, available follow-up care.
- If you are newly diagnosed, an allergist will help to educate you about what food allergies are, how they affect you, and what to look out for when you're having a reaction.
- If you've had food allergies a long time, an allergist will create an emergency plan with you, talk about how you will keep yourself safe in multiple scenarios, and test your current reaction severity.
- Don't be afraid to shop around to find a doctor who suits you best.

3

the reassurance room

After the first bite of pizza, my stomach felt hollow, my hands started to tingle, my mouth felt funny, and my throat—what was happening to my throat? Was it closing? Was it getting tight? Was I choking? Oh no, not here. Not with these people.

Everyone was drinking and smoking and being *molto gentile* (very nice). This was our last night in Venice. We had been here for two weeks, studying Italian in the morning, a few phrases of which I've retained: *Mi dispiace* is "I'm sorry," and *Dove* is "Where is." In the afternoon, we either drew with an artist in residence or went to see Titian and Tintoretto paintings with an art historian.

I was fifteen years old, on an art history tour of Italy. There were four other American teenagers; everyone else was English, in their gap year before going to university.

It was a pretty great trip, except for the eating part. I had my little card from the Italian consulate memorized: *niente noccioline* ("nothing with nuts"). I had been using it and had been sticking to the basics: eggs and white bread, pasta and tomato sauce, mozzarella and tomato panini, and a lot of mineral water.

That day I hadn't eaten much, and dinner was very late. By the time it came out, I was starved. Beyond starved; I was famished. And concerned. Perhaps I hadn't impressed upon my server the seriousness of my food allergies. (I hadn't wanted to make a scene, with the cool English boys nearby.) I wasn't wearing a medical alert bracelet (it hadn't been prescribed to me), and no autoinjectors of epinephrine were in my purse (no one was giving out prescriptions in the 1980s). It was just me and my heightened state of food awareness.

After just one bite of that stupid pizza, I knew something was terribly wrong. It had looked safe enough. It was a pizza Margherita: tomato sauce, fresh mozzarella, fresh basil, olive oil, and salt and pepper on a white-flour crust. It was named after a queen of Italy, and it was the plainest thing on the menu. No nuts, no fish. Common sense told me it was probably fine. But whom could I ask? My tablemates would have thought I was crazy. The Italian server? No luck there; he didn't speak English. "*Mi scusi, parlo solo Italiano,*" he said.

I looked around the table again. No one was looking at me; no one saw the fear on my face, the panic in my eyes. I felt as though I were watching myself at this dinner, hovering over the table, detached. Before I knew it, I was getting up, squeezing out of my cramped seat, pushing chairs aside, and running away from the group. There were some looks as I stood up, and perhaps a few people even called out to me in confusion or concern as I dashed from the table, knocking over chairs to get out.

The tape in my head screamed, "Get back to the *pensione*! Don't let anyone know!"

I ran through the streets of Venice toward the *pensione*, which was near the Santa Maria della Salute church. I had walked this route every day for a week now; I knew it by heart, even in a blind panic. I was running past piazzas and over *ponti* (bridges), past the expensive shops like Armani and Krizia, which I had just been browsing in an hour earlier; past the *ragazzi* (boys) in the Piazza San Marco, who shouted after me, "*Bella, bella!*"

All the while I was running, I was doing a body scan: Was I wheezing? Was I itchy? What was going on with my throat? With every step I tried to detect a new symptom of an allergic reaction. My hands were cramped. Was I hyperventilating? Was I anaphylaxing? Each step closer to the *pensione* was a step closer to being safe. Seven minutes of running, then ten; closer and closer. The streets became darker, quieter, fewer people and more trees; patches of dark blue summer sky emerged, and the Big Dipper hung sweet and low.

I slowed down near the Peggy Guggenheim museum. In the corner between the entrance to her house and the path to the next *pont* and toward safety, I realized that I had no hives and I wasn't wheezing. My lips weren't swollen, and my tongue seemed to be its normal size. My throat hadn't closed; I had been breathing and swallowing just fine.

I wasn't haven't a food-allergic reaction at all. I was having a panic attack.

food allergies and anxiety

Palpitations, shortness of breath, tingling hands, feeling detached, thinking I might go crazy or die, now I know those are the classic symptoms of a panic attack. According to the *Diagnostic and Statistical Manual of Mental Disorders*, a panic attack is a "discrete period of intense fear or discomfort, in which four (or more) of the following symptoms developed abruptly and reached a peak within 10 minutes: Palpitations, pounding heart, or accelerated heart rate; sweating; trembling or shaking; sensations of shortness of breath or smothering; feeling of choking; chest pain or discomfort; nausea or abdominal distress; feeling dizzy, unsteady, lightheaded, or faint; derealization (feelings of unreality) or depersonalization (being detached from oneself); fear of losing control or going crazy; fear of dying; numbness or tingling sensations; chills or hot flushes."

I experienced four or more of those symptoms, and the situation resolved within ten minutes or so. Textbook.

Living a food-allergic life, I've experienced many anxious moments. I'm not alone in these feelings. Those of us with severe food allergies can be an anxious group. This is something your allergist might not know, recognize, talk to you about, or know how to treat. However, it's real. I've heard it from too many of you and have felt it myself too often not to address it head-on.

The lingering anxiety around social events, holidays, dining out, dating, hanging out with friends, traveling—it's all there. Many of us struggle with food-allergy anxiety throughout our lifetimes, and some of us never resolve it. We avoid it, ignore it, or deny it, but we don't resolve the anxiety that comes with having a restricted diet because of food that causes uncomfortable and scary symptoms.

We're going to tackle those feelings in this chapter in an effort to give you some relief, some knowledge that you are not alone in these feelings, that they are normal and you can move through them.

tools for the newly diagnosed

If you have been diagnosed with a food allergy as an adult, you may have a wide range of reactions, ranging from disbelief to fear, depression, denial, and relief. Common feelings include the following:

- *Shame.* Feeling as though something is profoundly wrong with you that is deeply unfixable.
- *Embarrassment.* A reaction to experiencing the feelings of shame.
- *Confusion.* Wondering how food could make you so ill.
- *Worry.* Anticipating the next reaction.
- *Anxiety or panic.* Feeling more than worried; experiencing food allergy–like symptoms when eating foods to which you aren't actually allergic.
- *Depression.* Feeling weepy, angry, or low once you realize the far-reaching implications of not being able to eat whatever you want whenever you want.

All of these initial feelings can be alleviated through talking with the newest member of Team You, your allergist. Becoming educated about your diagnosis and knowing what to do in an emergency will greatly ease your mind. In addition, you can try the following simple activities:

- *Regular exercise.* A twenty-minute walk, running, biking, dancing in your living room, or dancing at a club—go, move.
- *Deep breathing.* Three deep, even breaths throughout the day can work small miracles.
- *Herbal teas or tisanes (infusions).* Mint, ginger, lavender, lemon verbena, and chamomile are some of my favorites.
- *Visualization.* I like an ocean scene; I immediately feel calm when I visualize one. Are you a mountain boy? A lake girl? Find your own happy, calm place and imagine you're there until your breath becomes even and soft.
- *Listening.* Treat your ears to something peaceful (classical music does it for me). Check out iTunes for easy listening, New Age, and meditation mixes galore.

- *Use of a mantra.* Try a word like *calm*, *free*, or *om*. Focus on that word as you breathe with your eyes closed. Try it for one minute. Build up to thirty minutes a day.
- *Meditation.* Find a free meditation group near you or download an iTunes meditation mix. Sit for a few minutes a day, eyes closed, and breathe deeply, letting your mind pulsate.
- *Other relaxation methods.* Supportive or alternative treatment modalities like acupuncture and/or a regular yoga practice can reduce feelings of generalized anxiety and the occasional panicky feelings.

Many of these tools are virtually free, and you have access to them any time you need them. Use them in nonanxious moments so you can call them up in an anxious moment.

Finding an outlet for your anxious feelings, a place to let them vent, is another vital component to anxiety management. This came from an Allergic Girl blog reader: "I had a very stupid accidental allergen exposure that landed me in my local emergency room. I've been suffering from panic attacks since then. I joined a support group and found there were a surprising number of us who developed panic attacks after a severe allergic reaction."

Support groups are excellent tools. Most local hospitals, community centers, religious centers, and mental health centers have them, and they are often free or very low-cost. Try one out or start your own. Talking with a friend or a loved one with whom you feel safe (see chapter 5), or consulting a food-allergy coach or other mental health professional for short-term work, will help you to move through these feelings about your food-allergy diagnosis.

it's okay to grieve

Once you've received an accurate food-allergy diagnosis, you may feel grief-stricken or be heartbroken over the change in your relationship to food. Perhaps you've heard about the stages of grief, sometimes referred to as the stages of dying. Dr. Elisabeth

Kübler-Ross wrote the seminal book *On Death and Dying* in 1969, in which she identified the five stages that most terminally ill patients experience:

* *Denial.* This isn't really happening.
* *Anger.* Why me? I don't deserve this!
* *Bargaining.* I'll do anything to make this go away.
* *Depression.* It's hopeless.
* *Acceptance.* This is who I am. I like myself, and I've accepted this part of me.

You don't have to be dying to experience these feelings or to travel along this arc of emotions. Any significant personal change that feels like a little death can elicit these stages of mourning. Recognize when you are experiencing these feelings so you can start to move through them. You can use grieving as an opening to a deeper conversation with yourself about your next steps.

How do you pass through these stages? How does anyone get to the end, to full acceptance? As someone who was aware she had food allergies practically from from day one, acceptance wasn't a process, it simply *was*. As the character Geordi La Forge of *Star Trek: The Next Generation* said when asked if he resented being blind, "Since it's a part of me and I really like who I am, there's no reason for me to resent it."

For those of you who are just coming to grips with a new diagnosis or are still moving along the spectrum of grief, getting there will happen naturally. It also happens in fits and starts; one moves back and forth along the spectrum of these feelings over time. There is no perfect timetable for going through grief and getting to the place of accepting your diagnosis and how food allergies will change your life. If you're a newly diagnosed food-allergic girl or guy, you may go back-and-forth through new feelings and emotions, some of them unpleasant and some uncomfortable, but all important to acknowledge and experience. Have patience with yourself and plenty of compassion.

listen to self-talk

Here's a simple exercise for knowing what you're feeling and when. Get quiet. Listen to the voice in your head. What is it whispering? What—a voice in your head? Do you even have that? Probably. We all engage in self-talk, even if we don't realize we're doing it. For example, the next time you're out to dinner, you might have a fleeting thought, a little voice that says, "A little of that allergen can't hurt me. I'll try just a bite or two. It'll be fine." This is classic denial. A little *can* hurt you; don't give in to it.

Recognizing self-talk takes time. Be patient. With practice you will be able to spot a negative thought a mile off. Once you can recognize a negative thought, you're halfway home. The next step, after recognizing that negative thought, is to reframe it as a positive or a realistic one. A reframed denial thought might sound like this: "I know a little of that allergen can hurt me. I want to stay safe, so I have taken the necessary precautions. I have my medications with me, I'm with friends I trust, and this restaurant is known to me. I'm okay." This gets easier with practice. Try. Practice.

being overly attuned

One step of the grieving process that's specific to the food-allergic experience is that of being overly sensitized, or overly attuned, to your body's functions. If you're too attuned, you can become paralyzed about eating everything; if you're not attuned enough, you can become glib about your health, ignoring obvious risks and dangers.

By necessity, food-allergic people have to be aware of bodily functions or changes. We need to stay aware of our bodies and how they may react to an allergen. Trouble develops when we perceive "Danger, Will Robinson" signals even when we've eaten something safe. Every throat tickle can feel like the beginning of the end; every stomach gurgle can send us flying into a panic. Symptoms become imagined, or tiny nuances of bodily functions are blown out of proportion.

Remember me at fifteen in Venice: a bite of pizza turned into a non–food allergic panic. I was overly attuned to my bodily functions and not tuned in to what was really happening in the present. Bodily awareness and being sensitive to any sudden change is critical; it keeps us safe. What can happen all too often, however, is that when we perceive danger from a potential allergen, we self-trigger a typical panicky fight-or-flight response.

The body's fight-or-flight response, the flooding of the body with adrenaline in order to defeat or flee from an enemy, is a highly evolved physiological response. The chemical cascade of natural adrenaline can make you feel jumpy, jittery, nervous, and anxious. Anxiety can appear to be an allergy feeling (closing throat, dry mouth, tingling extremities, sense of doom), which then leads us to feel allergic even when we are not. The main difference is that a panic attack will dissipate in about ten minutes, whereas an allergic reaction will (typically) worsen in the same amount of time. It's crucial to confer with your medical Team You about the difference between the symptoms of an allergic reaction and those of panic.

The trick is to be able to distinguish real responses from imaginary ones and real threats from perceived threats, and then be able

dealing with anxiety

If anxiety is paralyzing you, consider an evaluation from a qualified mental health professional affiliated with any of these reliable organizations:

A social worker (MSW)—National Association of Social Workers: www.socialworkers.org

A psychologist (PhD)—American Psychological Association: www.apa.org

A psychiatrist (MD)—American Psychiatric Association: www.psych.org

For more resources—National Institute of Mental Health: www.nimh.nih.gov/index.shtml

to contain your fear so it remains a survival skill but not a drain on your life. The goal is to honor fear as a useful tool in keeping you safe but not let it take over and paralyze you.

getting spooked isn't only for halloween

It was the birthday of my friend's husband, so my friend put together a lavish dinner at their large home. The event was catered by a chef who was given a heads-up about my food allergies by the hostess. When I arrived, the chef was preparing the dinner, and I was able to talk directly with him about the menu. He was making beet and goat cheese salad with hazelnuts and hazelnut oil for an appetizer and fish for the main dish. I saw the beets preroasted, sliced, and prepped on the kitchen counter.

"We'll make a separate plate for you without any hazelnuts or hazelnut oil," the chef said. In my mind that salad was already tagged as a no-go. It was too scary; too easy to have a mix-up or a "tainted" utensil involved. After the hors d'oeuvres were passed around and there were toasts with clinking glasses, we sat down at the table, and the appetizer was served.

My plate was indeed different: simple slices of roasted beet arranged prettily and glistening—in oil. What kind of oil did the chef end up using? I felt too embarrassed to ask, because he had already said it would be safe for me. But it didn't look safe; that oil could have been anything. I simply couldn't bring myself to eat it. I asked the guest to my right to taste it for the offending and frightening oil. He said it was just olive oil, but still, I couldn't bring myself to eat it. I was officially spooked.

Even if the salad was fine, and it probably was, I knew I wasn't going to enjoy it. So I skipped it; I left it untouched on my plate. I felt a little embarrassed and a little irrational, but I also knew, from years of experience, that if I ate the beet salad, I probably would've had a panicky moment imagining an allergic response.

(Yes, you can do that.) It's all a head trip, but it's no fun, and it would've made me miserable. My dinner companions on both sides of me ate my beet salad.

Next up was broiled chicken and asparagus risotto (completely different from the salmon being served all around me). My two adjacent dinner companions offered to taste it for me (so sweet of them). I said, "No thanks," instead pushing through my irrational fears and eating my delicious dinner. It was perfectly safe, and I felt better for not having let my fear get the better of me.

This dinner party was a lifetime away from that dinner party in Venice when I was fifteen. I was still spooked; however, I did not detach from the experience and run away. I communicated clearly, early and often to ensure my dining safety. My hostess was informed of my needs, the chef was informed of my needs, and I spoke directly with him as well. I listened to my internal voice, recognizing when I didn't feel safe. I did not judge those feelings, but honored them. I created dining allies on the spot (the two gentlemen sitting next to me who became my de facto food tasters). Best of all, because I had put all of those structures in place, when the second course came, I felt confident about dining, having honored and worked through my irrational fears.

Perhaps I should be "over this" by now, especially after a lifetime of daily practice. But I respect that sometimes getting spooked still happens. I know that if still happens to me, it can happen to you. Welcome to the sometimes-I-feel-panicky-when-I-eat food-allergic club.

the trauma of a reaction

Food is a sensory experience. Literature has exalted it; science has confirmed it. Gastronomic experts have quantified five flavors that our taste buds universally recognize: sweet, salty, sour, bitter, and umami (or savory). As animals, we are programmed to recognize poisonous tastes and spit out the offending food. This is natural. What also seems to be natural is that if we eat something to which we have an adverse or even scary reaction, we never want to eat it again.

Recall when you ate something and reacted to it with itchy lips, itchy ears, an itchy throat, hives, wheezing or a closing throat. Whatever set off the allergic chain reaction in your body, whether hidden pine nuts in a pesto or a secret fish sauce in the stir-fry, it's natural for you to want to avoid the food that hurt you. However, beyond an occasional anxious moment or an infrequent panicky feeling may be a persistent underlying fear that holds you back from living a fully realized life with food allergies. That underlying and nagging fear could be trauma.

Having a swift and severe reaction to a food, feeling your throat close up, needing emergency medication, or going to the emergency room are traumatic events. Something happens to the body, the mind, and the spirit after a really scary event: this is trauma. Everyone reacts to scary life events differently. For some people, a severe allergic reaction won't throw them. They discover the allergy, get the medications, and successfully avoid the allergen, with little disruption to their lives.

For others, the experience will stop them and paralyze them. Who can blame them? After a trauma like going to the hospital to be pumped full of lifesaving meds after eating something seemingly innocuous like shrimp scampi, when you had no previous adverse shrimp reactions, it's normal to be on high alert after the incident. A week, a few weeks, and maybe even a month or two is an average emotional reaction.

When high alert lasts beyond days or weeks and lingers for months or even years, you may be dealing with trauma. You might see and feel danger everywhere. A shrimp allergy becomes an imagined allergy to all shellfish, then all seafood. This can curtail your full enjoyment of life, friends, and normal activities like eating a balanced diet and enjoying your food. You've officially entered a trauma zone.

Most of us who've had a severe food-allergic reaction have had moments of feeling traumatized. However, if even *reading* about an itchy or scratchy throat, itchy ears, hives, a flushed feeling, the throat closing, the tongue swelling, a shortness of breath, or no breathing at all make you uneasy (that is, you almost feel those symptoms as you read about them), there is probably something deeper going on.

what exactly is trauma?

We've all heard the word *trauma* thrown around; watch any prime-time television medical or police drama, and trauma is everywhere. But what does it mean? Do you have it? How do you know when you've experienced it? According to Merriam-Webster's dictionary, the word *trauma* is derived from the Greek *titrōskein*, "to wound." A trauma represents a physical or a psychological wounding. MedicineNet.com defines this wounding as "a normal response to an extreme event. It involves the creation of emotional memories about the distressful event that are stored in structures deep within the brain. In general, it is believed that the more direct the exposure to the traumatic event, the higher the risk for emotional harm."

For many food-allergic individuals, this means that whether or not we've realized it, having a severe allergic reaction to a food may have created a deeply negative emotional memory tied to that reaction and subsequently to that food. This is food-allergy trauma.

Putting a name to something can be the first step in knowing the thing or, in this case, the feeling. I'm suggesting that we name the whole feeling group: all of those negative memories, the overwhelming and constant worry that it might happen again, the movie playing in your head of a severe allergic reaction happening again and again, the dreams (or nightmares) about another severe food-allergic event. All of this is trauma.

Naming a diagnosis, a feeling, or a symptom is a useful tool. But it is simply that: a tool. Names don't define us; they help to describe conditions that may affect us. Assigning a name to a condition, a diagnosis, a feeling, or a symptom should feel freeing, not more restrictive. Calling an anaphylactic event a trauma begins to quantify what happens every time you come into contact with the cause of that event—that is, the offending food.

Nevertheless, names or labels are not for everyone. The philosopher Søren Kierkegaard said, "Once you label me, you negate me." He was not fond of labels, and you may agree with him, being opposed to labeling your feelings after a severe food-allergic reaction as trauma. That's okay. Whatever you call it (or don't), it is vital to recognize that something is happening that may be interfering with your normal life functioning and/or adding to your life's burden.

Name it, don't name it—but *do not ignore it*. If you do ignore these feelings, you may end up with only one coping strategy: avoidance. Although avoidance is very effective and shouldn't be discarded from your toolbox, there are other coping strategies to add.

when the fear lingers

Those who have experienced at least one severe allergic reaction can experience deeper lingering feelings, nagging thoughts, unshakable irrational fears, and anxieties above and beyond those of a traumatic event. Individuals who have had multiple severe allergic reactions sometimes experience more than trauma and enter the state of post-traumatic stress disorder.

An Allergicgirl.com blog reader said:

> Up until four years ago, I was completely unaware I had any food allergies—until I had an anaphylactic attack. Some days I wake up and think the universe is playing a joke on me; some days I feel overwhelmed and have

panic attacks from fear of eating anything that might cause an allergic reaction. My GP calls it post-traumatic stress from the anaphylactic attack. All I know is that I'm scared all of the time!

Post-traumatic stress disorder (PTSD) is a big, scary term. It's also a big, scary set of feelings. In the past decade, PTSD has entered the zeitgeist with more alacrity than it has in years past, probably because so many of our young men and women in the armed forces are returning from a war zone after multiple tours of duty. The kind of PTSD a soldier experiences is different from what a food-allergic survivor faces; however, many of the features are similar.

MedicineNet.com describes PTSD as follows: "PTSD sufferers re-experience the traumatic event or events in some way, tend to avoid places, people, or other things that remind them of the event (avoidance), and are exquisitely sensitive to normal life experiences (hyperarousal)."

There are three groups of symptoms that are required for a diagnosis of PTSD:

1. Recurrent reexperiencing of the trauma, through troublesome memories or flashbacks that are usually caused by reminders of the trauma, recurring nightmares about the trauma, and/or dissociative reliving of the trauma
2. Avoidance to the point of having a phobia of places, people, and experiences that remind the sufferer of the trauma and a general numbing of emotional responsiveness
3. Chronic physical signs of hyperarousal, including sleep problems, trouble concentrating, irritability, anger, blackouts or difficulty remembering things, an increased tendency to being startled, and hypervigilance to threat.

After a severe food-allergic event, you may temporarily experience symptoms consistent with PTSD. The problem is when these temporary symptoms don't go away quickly, you don't normalize and feel like your old self again; or when the symptoms interfere with your daily functioning, sleeping, eating, living, and loving. If you experience any of these feelings or symptoms longer than a month, seek the guidance of a professional who has worked with trauma in all its forms to help you to move through the trauma to acceptance.

reacting to your reactions

Here's the challenge. Think about the following questions:

- How do you move forward, beyond the fear, beyond the phobia, beyond the routine that you have prescribed for yourself up until now?
- How do you protect yourself while still living your life fully?
- How do you ever feel safe again?
- How do you ever trust your body after it has betrayed you by being allergic?
- How do you avoid food without avoiding food?
- How do you build new positive relationships with food?
- How do you change the voice inside your head, a voice you maybe didn't even realize you had?
- How do you think about food allergies in a new and positive way?
- How do you build new positive experiences with food when you're dining out, traveling, or eating with friends, family, or your romantic partner?

This is what we are going to explore. I'm going to help you own this diagnosis, make it yours, and take it seriously and then help others to take it seriously as well. We are not going to eliminate fear—fear is good and healthy and normal—but we are going to keep fear in check as we move forward.

allergic girl's reassurances

- When you first receive a food-allergy diagnosis, you may feel embarrassed, ashamed, worried, confused, or depressed. This is normal.
- In conjunction with a board-certified allergist, educate yourself about your food-allergic reality versus your fears and work through your feelings.
- Remember, you are not alone if you feel anxious from time to time about food allergies or a potential food-allergic reaction.
- For low-level anxiety, stress-busting activities (such as yoga, exercise, and meditation) work well, are easy to do, and are often free or at least low-cost.
- For lingering anxiety after a severe food-allergic reaction, support groups are an excellent outlet; so is talking with understanding friends, family, and your romantic partner.
- Many people who receive a food-allergy diagnosis go through the steps of deep grieving. This is normal. Allow yourself to travel along the spectrum of feelings toward acceptance.
- As you travel along that spectrum, recognize when you engage in injurious self-talk, then reframe those statements as positive ones.
- If anxiety or feelings of panic linger, interrupt normal daily functioning, or paralyze you, or if you find that you are stuck in the trauma of a food-allergic reaction and cannot move past it, seek support from a qualified mental health practitioner.

part two

relationships

4

nothing to prove

When you love them they drive you
crazy because they know they can.

—Rose Castorini, *Moonstruck*

T hat doesn't look right."

"You're right. What are those brown bits?"

"I have no idea, but I don't think I should eat it. Would you taste it for me?"

After scooping up a small spoonful of ice cream and tasting the brown bits, my mother said, "They're hazelnuts! Let's get the server."

We were at a café in the heart of Little Italy in New York City. I was thirteen years old. The café is a classic; it's been there since the late 1890s. The owners make their own breads, cakes, and cookies in the bakery next door. When you leave and walk to the right, the odor of fresh yeast wafts and wheat flour plumes. It's heavenly. Inside, the café has retained its vintage pressed tin ceilings, ice cream parlor chairs, marble tabletops, and a picture window overlooking the foot traffic.

My mother and I visited this café regularly for decaffeinated cappuccinos and nut-free cookies. On this night I had altered the usual routine and ordered vanilla ice cream instead. When it arrived, my food-allergic instinct said that I shouldn't eat it. I was self-trained to always look at everything I ate; I rarely just popped something into my mouth. (I did that once in my life and learned my lesson. See chapter 1.) My mom offered to taste it for me. When I was little, my mother offered to taste things to reassure me that nothing was wrong and that the food was safe to eat. It wasn't until I was older that she said, "I can't really distinguish the ingredients in your dish." As a teen, I still asked her from time to time to taste something (and even now, as a thirty-something year old).

My mother and her taste testing definitely helped with a few narrow escapes. She was with me for scores of food-allergic reactions, some scary and some necessitating a hospital visit, some in restaurants and some at friends' houses. On this night, because I had ordered vanilla ice cream with nothing on it and it came with conspicuous flecks that shouldn't be in vanilla, tasting definitely seemed in order.

The server confirmed that there were hazelnuts in the vanilla ice cream and said, without a hint of irony, "That's how we always make it." My mother became irate, as any parent would. "If your vanilla ice cream contains nuts, then that should be listed on the menu. My child is allergic, and if she had eaten this, she would have gotten severely ill." The server simply shrugged and asked if we'd like something else. We were too upset to eat, however, and I was feeling generally unsafe, so we left. We would go back for decaffeinated cappuccinos and nut-free cookies, but I would never order ice cream again.

In terms of my food allergies, my mother has always been my supporter, protector, nurturer, champion, and advocate. Our apartment, I realize in hindsight, was an Allergic Girl haven. Everything was Sloane-safe. There was never an argument or a debate, never a blame-game or a guilt-trip; it was just a state of being. It wasn't until I came home from college and saw some nuts on the kitchen counter and fish in the fridge that I realized how many foods she had given up to make our home safe. Ah, family.

the importance of family acceptance

Full acceptance of your food-allergy diagnosis is essential if you are to move through a food-allergic life confidently, with ease and joy. Understanding what a food allergy is and how it affects you, having a medical Team You with whom to confer about your diagnosis, and identifying your feelings will all help you to get to that level of acceptance. The next step is to get your family, your friends, and your romantic partners on board.

A family is a complicated, complex system of personalities, temperaments, and characters. Families come in all shapes, sizes, and structures. Parents can be biological, adopted, foster, or chosen. They can be whoever took care of you as a child, nurtured you, and protected you; whoever you consider your biggest fans and biggest supporters; and whoever would have been your food taster. Having a family that gets it (whether immediately or with some assistance from you) will help you to reach the golden zone of full acceptance of your food-allergic diagnosis and your food-allergic lifestyle needs.

Families respond differently when one of their members receives a potentially life-threatening medical diagnosis. Some families will take up the cause immediately, the majority will need a period of adjustment, and some families (or extended family members) may never quite understand. Let's walk through specific examples of each type of family.

Families That Take Up the Cause

Whether you were diagnosed a long time ago or recently, some families take up your dietary restrictions with gusto. The members of such a family will educate themselves on what you need and how they can help; they will read books, do research online for reliable information, and find or start support groups. They can become your best advocates.

Elizabeth Landau, a CNN.com writer who's allergic to tree nuts, peanuts, artichokes, and seafood, told me this about her mom:

> If there's anyone determined to make sure that I eat safely, it's my mom. My mom would never offer me peanut butter without thinking, or forget to read the ingredients on a package of cookies. Since I first started having bad reactions to certain foods as a child, she became my advocate in making sure that everything I ate was safe. I have heard of some parents separating "safe" foods from "unsafe" foods in the pantry, but we just eliminated peanuts and nuts from the kitchen altogether. "It's not that great," my mom would always say if she ate something that might have been cross-contaminated. . . . These days, when I go home to visit and we go out to eat, she'll still quiz me about whether I'm sure I can eat whatever it is I want to order. I'm an adult now and can make my own decisions, but it's good to know that there's still someone looking out for me.

Jennifer Kales of nut-freemom.blogspot.com said this about her child's grandparents:

> My mom made her house nut-free as soon as she found out about my daughter's allergy. She's extremely careful.

My sister also went nut-free and asks me about foods and provides the safe ones each time we visit. She is 100% for her niece. Before every visit, my mother-in-law asks me about ingredients and foods. She's a great cook and told me at our last visit that she appreciated eating and preparing "good simple food" when we visit.

Cathy, a Worry-Free Dinners family member, told me this story about how her family deals with her son Nick's food allergies:

The one person [who] has been the biggest positive influence in Nick's life has been my mother, MaryJane. We were living with my parents when Nick was born. Both my husband and I worked full-time, and she stayed with him all day. When he was nine months old she fed him macaroni and cheese baby food. Twenty minutes later he was vomiting, hives [had erupted] all over his body, and saliva was running out of his mouth. She had no idea what was happening. I pulled into the driveway as she was leaving to take him to the doctor. That was his first anaphylactic reaction. We discovered Nick is allergic to dairy, eggs, peanuts, and tree nuts.

From that day on she was determined to make his life as normal as possible, including redesigning the traditional Italian meatball and making special holiday cookies with a margarine that is safe for him. She has a summer home at the beach where our three families go and spend summers; it's a large group. She rearranged her whole kitchen so that he would have his own refrigerator, microwave, and snack baskets. Taking my mother's lead, my entire family has acclimated themselves to knowing that keeping Nick safe is the most important thing when we are together. His cousins are diligent about hand washing and only eating snacks that are safe for him.

About six summers ago, my brother suggested that everyone in the house—family, nannies and guests—be trained on how to use the Epi-Pen. He wanted to know where [it] would be located and for everyone to know how to get to the hospital. I was floored. I would always randomly show my sister-in-law and nannies how to use the Epi-Pen, but this was great. And now we do it every year.

Food-allergic adult, new mother, and Allergicgirl.com blog reader Jess told me this about her father and brother:

I had to be on bed rest for part of the pregnancy, and other people had to do food shopping for me. My father, who owns a consulting company, and my brother came up with an application for his mobile phone that had lists of the foods to which I was allergic and the synonyms for them. He gave this app to the people in my family who were doing my food shopping, which really helped. I thought it was so great and helpful that they turned it into a free application for the iPhone.

Millions of families are like these, motivated and acting decisively when confronted with an adult child's, a young child's, or a grandchild's food-allergy diagnosis. Some families have even taken it to the next step, creating advocacy forums, nonprofit organizations, "Don't feed me my allergen" clothing and apparel companies, smart phone applications, and food-manufacturing companies for their food-allergic loved ones.

The Food Allergy and Anaphylaxis Network, for instance, was started by the mother of a food-allergic child, and so was the Food Allergy Initiative. Cherrybrook Kitchen was created by a food-allergic adult, Enjoy Life Foods was founded by the son of a food-allergic mother, and Divvies: Made to Share goodies was started by the parents of a food-allergic child.

If this is your kind of family, you are one lucky duck. Education, patience, and awareness are the keys to helping your family to keep helping you. Don't forget to let them know how much you appreciate their efforts and the ways in which they can continue the great work. Notes, e-mails, cards or electronic cards, and pleases and thank-yous are all appreciated.

Send a thank-you note to your family? Shouldn't your family members just normally do these things for you? Perhaps, but that doesn't mean you shouldn't still be appreciative; that's part of the love equation. Let the family members who do a great food-allergy job know that you love and appreciate them; it will encourage them to keep doing it.

For example, my first cousin Gregg and his wife, Lynn, host Thanksgiving. A week before, Lynn gets in touch with me and we go over the menu. She tells me what she's making and who is bringing what. I tell her what I'll probably be eating and bringing so she can plan for any nutty dishes, if she wishes. The resulting dinner is a buffet, which is delicious and Sloane-safe. (I make sure to get in line early to avoid "contaminated" spoons. See chapter 10 for more strategies.)

The day after, I send my cousins an e-mail to let them know that their hard work was appreciated and did not go unnoticed: "Dear Lynn and Gregg, Thank you both for a lovely Thanksgiving evening. It was delish, safe, and fun. Love you, Sloane."

I once asked Lynn how she makes it all so easy. She said it's because I've talked to her about my food allergies, I've let her know my needs ahead of time, and she understands that it's simply a fact of life. She's happy to make accommodations so I can partake. Some extended family members will be happy to get on board the food-allergy train.

Bonus: Spread the love. Be an ally for another family member. Has someone else gotten a medical diagnosis recently or gone through a rough patch? Take the support you receive and "pay it forward" to the next family member who needs it. Be supportive, kind, understanding, and accommodating; go out of your way to assist, lend an ear or a shoulder, or help in whatever way he or she needs.

Families That Need Time to Adjust

From my food-allergy coaching practice, I know that most families will need a period of adjustment. Just as you may have done, your family members may need to go through the stages of grief once they learn about your food-allergy diagnosis. They may linger over negative feelings as they pass through the stages: denial, anger, bargaining, depression, and acceptance. Everyone's acceptance of your diagnosis is the goal, the target to work toward.

Adjustment to a new diagnosis often involves innocent food mistakes, as in this story from Terri, a food service industry colleague and the mother of a peanut-allergic child:

> Brad was two when he was diagnosed with a severe peanut allergy. From that moment on, we read all food labels and questioned servers in restaurants before we allowed him to ingest any food. When Brad was seven, we went to Vermont to see the foliage. One day, we were in a country store, and there were jars of spreads with crackers for sampling. We confidently sampled an apple butter, after reading the label, and moved to the next item, which was a maple spread.
>
> After putting the light-brown spread on a cracker, I started to read the ingredients. Simultaneously, I gave the sample to Brad, which he put promptly in his mouth. I usually read the ingredients first; however, this time I did not. The first listed ingredient was peanut butter! I looked at Brad, who had already put the cracker in his mouth and was chewing, and I said sternly, "Don't swallow." He immediately opened his mouth and began to gag from fear, as I whisked him off to the restroom, where he got rid of what was left.

Fortunately, there was no reaction, and we dodged the bullet. It was such a staggering experience for us both. I was overly confident and put Brad in harm's way; he lost his confidence in me for a short time. Although we question everything before he puts anything unfamiliar in his mouth, it was a good exercise, since we learned that we can never let our guard down.

Heidi, the mother of a food-allergic child and the head of a parents' food-allergy support group, told me this story:

We've developed our strategy over the past twelve years and perfected it. Except when Grandma visits, and then our normally well-controlled food-allergic kitchen becomes confusing and chaotic. Within moments of arriving in the kitchen, Grandma has spoons dipping into allergen-laden sauces and [has] quickly mixed [them] with our child's safe dish. Dishes are poorly washed with contaminated sponges, leaving my husband and I to merely gasp. Though Grandma means well, her presence and inability to sit idly by while we do the cooking is a source of incredible stress for us.

Worry-Free Dinners family members Mike and Tara are the parents of Ava, a severely peanut-allergic child. Mike told me this about their family:

Tara's parents did a lot of obvious things as soon as we found out about Ava's allergy (put the peanut butter on a high shelf whenever we were visiting, for example) but didn't really grasp that when they were going to be around her and kiss her, they really needed to be cognizant of what they were putting in their own mouths [and] to be diligent about washing up, etc. One day, Tara's dad kissed Ava on the arm after coming from a fast-food restaurant where he had not eaten peanuts but must have been exposed to something—she got hives right away. The fact that that happened made him so upset with himself that he won't even go near her without washing up first, just in case he has eaten something peanut-y without realizing it.

This is all a normal part of a family's adjustment.

A medical diagnosis that requires the whole family to shift for one member can be demanding. Heidi told me this story about how her family wants to understand but chooses an inappropriate time to have the talk:

> The other unique phenomenon that happens with Grandma, and many other family members, is that they're never quite sure what our daughter's allergies are. And instead of asking before they visit, they like to make it into an hour-long discussion, which is uncomfortable for us and for them. We try to limit those conversations when at all possible and deflect [them] with sentences like "She's thirteen now and has an exemplary diet, is right on track for weight and height, and is very intelligent.

Invariably, food allergies require major adjustments for an entire household, including the possible elimination of a favorite ingredient. The need to eliminate some old favorite foods may push some family members temporarily off the "happy ship." For example, Mike (of Mike and Tara) told me the following story:

> One of my aunts is an avid baker. Usually, she bakes all of the Christmas cookies for Christmas Eve—about 10 different varieties in all, including peanut butter balls. Initially, she would usually bake all of these cookies together on the same day. She stopped making them because no one wanted to worry about whether or not

any peanut butter crossed with another butter cookie. We commended her for giving up that long-standing tradition without a grudge, but [we] were hopeful we could make her comfortable baking again.

At first, she didn't understand why cocoa that isn't marked as being manufactured around nuts might nonetheless have been, and that got frustrating. However, we recently introduced her to a peanut-free chocolate, and her confidence in being able to bake safely has increased. Last weekend, she made a safe allergen-free chocolate cake for my brother's birthday that we could all enjoy.

Your job is to help your family get back on the "happy ship," just as you are working through your feelings, too.

Families That Don't Get It

Every food allergic adult has someone, or several someones, in the family who refuse to get the whole "food-allergy thing." It may be the uncle who calls you the "boy in the bubble," the cousin who rolls her eyes when you bring special food to a family gathering, a sister who still sends you peanut brittle on your birthday even though she knows you're severely peanut-allergic, a mother who apologizes for your "picky eating habits" to servers when you're dining out, or an aunt who forwards you online articles about "miracle" allergy cures. Jibes, nonverbal digs, and misunderstandings about the nature of food allergies can leave you feeling like a difficult, high-maintenance, annoying, and unloved family member.

Families have a tremendous power to hurt one's feelings. This is not particular to the food-allergic community; it's global. Know this: When it comes to your food allergies, you have nothing to prove. Once you realize that you have nothing to prove, you will:

- Be set free from family drama about your food-allergy diagnosis

- See that your food allergies are not up for negotiation
- Take your health and your dietary needs out of other people's hands and put them back into your own

It's natural for a family member with a difference, such as a medical diagnosis, to be singled out. With family members you see less often or are less close to, there can be more confusion, cluelessness, and misapprehension of crucial details. There may be provocative, impolite, and unsympathetic comments made about your dietary needs. Families can be insensitive, and they can be oblivious to the psychological damage that a seemingly innocent question can incur. How to manage insensitive statements takes practice, but it is possible to move past the verbal jabs and punches and access the love that your family offers.

support yourself as you support your family

It's a big task, I know: helping them, helping yourself, helping them to help you. This is another reason it's vital that you have clarity about your diagnosis, how to treat it, and what to do in an emergency. Go back and read the first section of the book for more support. If you feel in need of even more assistance—and that would be very natural—go to your board-certified allergist or internist for a chat, hire a food-allergy coach, join a support group or create one, go to an online forum, and read food-allergy blogs, magazines, and books. At the very least, reach out and work through your food-allergy diagnosis so you can help your family to accept this part of you.

mike and celiac disease

You may be surprised how deep your family's relationship to food is and how unwilling they are to give up certain foods so you can be safe when you're with them. As Grace Adler from TV's *Will & Grace* said, "Jews and chicken . . . it's real and it's deep." Truer words were rarely spoken. Let's look at how coaching client Mike handled his medical diagnosis and his new life with dietary restrictions.

Mike is twenty-four years old. A recent college graduate, he's living at home in upstate New York while working as an information technology engineer for a large corporation. He sought coaching to help him cope with his medical diagnosis. After a visit to a knowledgeable gastroenterologist and several tests, he uncovered the medical reason for years of unexplained stomach problems: celiac disease.

Celiac disease is not a food allergy; it is a genetic autoimmune disease in which gluten cannot be ingested (gluten is the protein found in wheat, barley, and rye). Exposure to gluten can incur severe discomfort in the short run and serious autoimmune system complications in the long run. The only cure for celiac disease is a strictly restricted diet: no gluten in any form. When Mike consumes gluten, he becomes gassy, is uncomfortably bloated, and has diarrhea for three days. He has spent much of his life running to the bathroom, feeling awkward in social situations and being generally unwell most of the time.

Mike is from a large Italian American family. After his celiac disease diagnosis, his five siblings and his parents were tested, too, because celiac disease is genetic. Two of Mike's younger siblings

celiac disease

Celiac disease, as defined by the Celiac Disease Center at Columbia University, is "an autoimmune disorder that causes damage to the small intestine, which can lead to malabsorption of nutrients."

have the disease but are asymptomatic; his mother doesn't have it, but his father does. The family's preferred diet is wheat-based: sandwiches, pizza, and big Sunday dinners of pasta. Mike's Italian grandmother, Nona, cooks her famous gravy and macaroni every week, but now that three kids and Dad cannot have gluten, the whole house has to be gluten-free.

Everyone feels the loss. One of Mike's younger siblings cheats regularly by sneaking pizza after school; another sibling eats bagged pretzels with school lunch. Dad is moody and sneaks doughnuts at the office, then comes home ill. Nona is completely flummoxed. She says, "It's just a little pasta, it can't possibly hurt anyone" as she ladles out her hand-rolled gnocchi. Mike doesn't want to hurt her feelings and is therefore conflicted about saying, "No, thanks, it will make me sick." (So instead he eats it and gets sick.)

Mom is overwhelmed with all of the family's dietary changes and is trying to cook for everyone safely but in a completely new way. The family budget is suffering from buying commercially made gluten-free foods that no one really likes. With so many members of the family in different stages of adjustment, the first few months after the celiac disease diagnosis have been chaotic.

During my phone sessions with Mike, we work together to help him manage his new gluten-free lifestyle. Through talking about his feelings of disappointment, confusion, anger, and relief that he finally knows what was going on with his digestive system, Mike was able to start the process of accepting his diagnosis. Part of that acceptance was feeling motivated to help the rest of the family. Through an online search, Mike discovered a celiac disease support group at the local hospital, and he suggested they all attend.

By going to the group, the family learned how other families were coping with their diagnoses, about the perils of cross-contamination and hidden gluten sources, and where to get less expensive gluten-free foods. They also connected with other celiac-disease families. They loved the group and became regular active members. They even found a gluten-free baking class at the neighboring culinary school, and Nona went there to learn how to make gluten-free doughnuts and gnocchi.

Within days of cutting out gluten from his diet, Mike felt an improvement; when he cheated, he immediately felt the repercussions. After three months of our work together, Mike's noticed some emotional respite. Working through his feelings about his and the family's diagnosis; utilizing local support; and creating new eating, cooking, and food-shopping patterns helped to normalize life for everyone. There would be mistakes, and there was the extended family to deal with, but now they could all see the path that leads to acceptance and health.

Adjustment is a natural process when someone is confronted with a massive life change, and there's no right or wrong timeline. It's not an overnight process. It will take time to move along the spectrum of grieving and the feelings of anger or resentment as a family makes the necessary adjustments. Worry-Free Dinners member Mike (of Mike and Tara) writes the following:

> Another example of someone acting without thinking is an uncle who was visiting our shore house for the weekend who brought a flat of muffins that included banana nut, and chips that were clearly marked as possibly containing peanuts. We tend to get very polarized by this, but have been trying to realize that it isn't an active slap in the face—these people just aren't living with it every day. We try to use those moments as teaching moments, and every week, month, year people seem to be more aware.

Your job is to keep moving forward as best as you can. Go back over certain steps when you need to, and check in with your friends, your doctors, and other members of Team You. Give yourself a break if you become angry, cheat on your gluten-free diet, or have an allergic reaction. You'll have another chance tomorrow to do better.

doing the zigzag

I spent years feeling hurt and indignant toward my extended family about holiday gatherings (see chapter 10). They forgot my needs, downplayed the seriousness of them, or just ignored them completely. I didn't see my extended family often, and because I have environmental allergies, asthma, and food allergies, there were a lot of details to get right. In hindsight, being indignant got me nowhere. The family members who didn't understand my allergic needs weren't suddenly enlightened because I was self-righteous. Hardly. All they understood was that Sloane is overly sensitive about allergies. And to be honest, I was overly sensitive. When I was a child, I lost years of extended family love. As an adult, it was time to try something new.

Life coach Martha Beck wrote about a technique for dealing with unkind statements. She calls it doing the zigzag. "[Mean people] expect a fight-or-flight reaction from their victims—either angry pushback or slinking away. The one thing they don't antici-pate is relaxed discernment. Scuttle their plans by zigging instead of zagging, cheerfully accepting any accurate statement they might make while ignoring their malicious energy." This is excellent gen-eral advice that I've adapted for the food-allergic community. The technique works exceptionally well, and I've coached scores of cli-ents to use it, with excellent results. When it's done well, the mean comment goes away and you're left with a positive connection to your interlocutor. It's a win-win.

Your task is to do the following:

- Depersonalize the insensitive comment, accept any grain of truth, and switch topics quickly. This will take practice. Help yourself by devising a few stock comebacks to draw upon at a moment's notice.
- Beware. There's a natural temptation to be all *pauvre moi* (poor me) here, to agree with the negative statement in a

way and thus justify it. Resist that urge; it will only drag you into a conversation that you can't win, and it may leave you feeling worse.

- Keep the situation positive; do not give anyone more ammunition by being self-deprecating.
- Deflect the attention; keep to the point and move on.

Following is some typical dialogue with two options. The first option is the self-righteous, defensive, self-deprecating "I'm hurt!" place you may feel like going to (or do go to) immediately; the second option is the detached, depersonalized, zigzag option. This is not about right or wrong; this is about creating options. When you're ready to try something new, give the second option a try. If it doesn't work the first time, keep finessing, keep fine-tuning, and keep trying until you find the right balance for you.

Family member 1: "I read that you can cure food allergies by taking pills. Why don't you just do that?"

Self-righteous option: "Pills—are you kidding me? You have no idea what you're talking about! There are no pills for this! Haven't I said it a million times? There is no cure!"

Detached option: "I'd love to be able to take a pill. If you remember the name of those pills, e-mail me. Speaking of e-mail, have you heard about the new applications Google.com is rolling out? Let me tell you more . . ."

Family member 2: "I heard that most people are just making food allergies up."

Defensive option: "Making this up? You think I want this? Who would ever want this? Why on earth would I do that?"

Depersonalized option: "Wouldn't it be fantastic if that were true? For me, food allergies are quite real and dangerous. Speaking of dangerous, is that outfit new? Watch out, here comes Aunt Bea, and *she's* dangerous!"

Family member 3: "You have so many food allergies, you really should just live in a bubble."

Self-deprecating option: "You're right. I know what a burden it is for you when I come over. Why do I even bother?"

Zigzag option: "I already have my safe bubble, being here with the family I love! By the way, the house looks really great. Did you finally get those curtains you wanted?"

When you're ready to let go, when you realize that some family members will just never get it, come up with your own snappy retorts to have on hand that are polite but that move on past an unwinnable topic. Remember: acknowledge, deflect, and move on. A compliment, in particular, will help you to move past the topic quickly. Everyone likes to hear nice things about himself or herself. Just make sure that it's sincere; no one likes a phony.

the shy zigzag

If you're a shy food-allergic person and feel unable or unwilling to say any of these direct retorts, that's fine. Find one of your bolder family members and make him or her your advocate or ally. It could be a parent, a sibling, a spouse, or a cousin—anyone who is sympathetic to your needs and doesn't feel shy. Identify that person, talk with him or her privately about your concerns, and create a signal to indicate when you need that person to come and help you.

Here's an example. "Aunt Susie, would you do me a favor? Aunt Bea keeps cornering me with stories she's seen on television about "food-allergy cures." I know she means well, but I feel trapped when she starts talking to me about this stuff. If you notice that she's cornered me, would you come and get me out of there? That would really help me out." If you're stuck in a food-allergy conversation that's going nowhere, you now have an easy and polite rescue.

If you have no allies within the family, or you haven't identified them yet, you can excuse yourself from the conversation just as you would do at any party. For example, if you're cornered by a well-meaning but misguided family member who wants to grill you about how "food allergies are all in your head," politely excuse yourself by saying that you need a drink refill or a bathroom visit; pretend you need more food or wave to an imaginary cousin and go talk to him or her.

Do what you need to do to leave a conversation that's going nowhere. Remember, you *never* have to stay and listen to an insensitive family member's theories on why you should just "get over" your food allergies.

release the wish

It's essential for your continued mental health to manage your expectations. Most family members will support you, but they might not be as exacting as you are, as clued in, or as allergy aware. Even after years of educating them and sending them books, news articles, and new research, and even when they've seen stories on television and in the newspaper, you may find that some family members never understand your food allergies or your needs.

If you've done everything you can to help them, it's time to release the wish for them to change. Release any need to be indignant or righteous about your food-allergic needs. Release the feeling that your family should automatically get it, that they should automatically understand and know how to support you. Releasing the wish is akin to disarmament. Once you release those deep wishes, the war will be over and you can accept all of the other loving aspects about your family.

allergic girl's family matters

- Some family members will understand immediately. Cherish this quality and let them know how much you appreciate their support.
- Most families need a period of adjustment in order to arrive at a place of acceptance about your food-allergic diagnosis.
- If you require assistance in adjusting and helping your family to adjust, consider seeking help in the form of short-term food-allergy coaching, local or online support groups, food-allergy books, talks with your allergist, or reputable online resources.
- Some families may not really understand. Manage your expectations with them and put your health first.
- Realizing that you have nothing to prove will help you to deal with family members who will never quite understand your food allergies.
- If you're shy, find an advocate within the family to help you with difficult family members.
- Releasing the wish for full acceptance from families that don't get it will help you to accept all the other love and support your family has to offer.

5

the loves of your life

You're the loves of her life, and a
guy's lucky if he comes in fourth.

—Mr. Big, *Sex and the City*

I've informally polled nearly everyone: friends from grade school, high school, college, and graduate school; and even brand-new friends, pre–and post–Allergicgirl.com blog. I've asked everyone the same question: Do you remember when I told you that I had food allergies? No one remembers having the food-allergy talk, but everyone knows that I have food allergies and fully accepts and supports this part of me.

So what's going on? Has everyone been struck by a sudden Best Friend Forever memory loss? No. Did they learn about my food allergies through osmosis? No. Was there a mass e-mail sent out about my food allergies? No. Do all of my friends also have food allergies, and we belong to some kind of secret sect of New Yorkers that I'm not telling you about? Really, no.

It's something deeper and more precious: the way that a true friend offers the kind of love that no other relationship can offer. The best friendships aren't hampered by a little something like food allergies. Friends, in many ways, are the loves of your life; friendship is a connection that is not bound by genetics or law. In the best scenario, friends are a fundamental component of your overall support system.

However, as my Omah (my other grandmother) said, "You have different friends for different things." So I hope you have some "loves of your life" friends (from whom you can create safe friends), and some inner- and outer-circle friends who will all get on board with your food-allergy diagnosis. Let's examine the functions your friends play when you're coping with a dietary restriction.

safe friends

Aimee and I have been friends since first grade. In every yearbook, we're side by side, laughing our heads off. We've gone through almost all of the life stages together, which now include food allergies. (Aimee has no allergies, but recently her youngest daughter, Kate, was diagnosed with allergic asthma, environmental allergies, and severe peanut allergies.)

Back in high school, weekends often included window shopping and then taking the nearby healing waters of frozen hot chocolate and pink lemonade. One afternoon, while I was home from college, I was with Aimee and another high school friend (who worshiped at the altar of the hot fudge sundae) for a revival of old high school times. Back then, I was an ovo-lacto vegetarian (that is, one who eats eggs and dairy but no meat or fish), so I ordered a veggie sandwich from the menu. I told our server about my tree-nut allergy, and he said there were no tree nuts in or on the sandwich.

When he brought me the veggie sandwich, though, I had a gut feeling that something was amiss. Before I ate it, I inspected it. The sandwich had an orange spread on both sides of the bread. It didn't say anything about a spread on the menu, so I didn't eat it. I asked Aimee if she would try it for me. Without a second thought, she took one swipe of the spread with her spoon. "That has almonds in it. Don't eat it!"

We called the server over, and he confirmed that there was an almond spread on the veggie sandwich. He seemed completely unconcerned that I had told him I was allergic to nuts and he served me something with nuts. All he did was to ask if I wanted something else. No, thanks. I finished my rather large pink drink and dined elsewhere. Thank goodness Aimee tasted it for me, though. Aimee was one of my safe friends.

I first identified some safe friends in high school, and I am happy to say that I had several options. These were the people to whom I could turn and be completely myself, even during high school, when self-consciousness about any difference can be overpowering. These friends—Aimee was on the top of that list and still is—were at heart the nonjudgmental, accepting sort. They understood that having food allergies is a medical need, that there could be an emergency situation, and that we might need to get help. They also understood that I was extra anxious about my food allergies and that there would be certain situations in which I would need extra understanding. It sounds like a lot for a teenager to deal with, and it was, but it was made so much each easier by having a safe friend.

Having one safe friend in your life can increase your joy multifold. Identifying or creating a safe person is a classic technique in cognitive-behavioral treatment for anxiety. It greatly reduces the burden of feeling scared and alone in an anxious or phobic-inducing situation. (You should remember however, that you are always your best first responder in an emergency situation.) For example, dining out somewhere new is often an anxious situation; doing it with a safe friend dramatically decreases that anxiety. With a safe friend, you may even be able to tackle a situation you deemed too scary to do solo, whether it's going for a food challenge at the doctor's office or practicing talking to a date about your needs.

A safe friend is usually a friend you've known a long time, so trust as well as a positive communication style have already been established. Whomever you believe to be safe is who's right for you, though, however long you have known him or her. Don't let a minor detail like length of time be the adjudicator in choosing a safe friend.

mike and his safe person

After Mike received his diagnosis of celiac disease (see chapter 4), for which the only cure is eliminating all gluten from one's diet, it wasn't only Mike's family that needed to adjust. Mike felt uncertain about how to broach the topic with his Monday night poker buddies. Their standard fare was a six-foot-long hoagie sandwich with copious amounts of beer (both full of gluten and thus off-limits for Mike).

Mike had learned that even a small bite of bread or a drop of beer would induce unbearable celiac disease symptoms for days. He wasn't going to stop going to poker night, but he wasn't ready to tell his buddies that he had "a disease." He ended up eating just the insides of the sandwich, but due to the contamination—the effect from the insides of the sandwich having just *touched* the bread—he was sick for more than three days.

This was not a great solution, as he felt more alone *and* symptomatic. In addition, his friends teased him about his many bathroom trips (symptoms of the disease). They weren't trying to be mean, but they had no idea what was going on, because Mike had hidden his diagnosis. Not normally a shy person, Mike suddenly felt very shy about talking about his needs with his friends.

In our coaching sessions, Mike and I explored the idea of identifying one person in whom he felt he could confide. He identified his best buddy, Dave, who was also at the poker nights. Mike and I practiced talking to Dave about his symptoms, what he was going through, and what he needed. We came up with five sentences that could accomplish this task efficiently: "Hey, Dave, I found out recently I have celiac disease. It's genetic, and it means I get sick and have to go to the bathroom when I eat anything with gluten, the protein in wheat, barley, and rye. So no more beer and sandwiches. I'm feeling weird about raising the issue with everyone else, but I wanted to tell you, since I knew you'd understand. I could really use an ally to help me figure out how to not get sick at poker night but still have a good time."

At the next poker night, Mike pulled Dave aside before the game and used the sentences we had practiced. Dave asked a few poignant questions, like what could Mike eat, said he was "totally cool" with it, and asked how he could help. Mike told me that he felt a great sense of relief knowing that at least one of his peers was on his side.

Mike and I explored more options, such as how he could talk to his other buddies, how he could manage his feelings in a social setting, and how he wanted to move forward. Mike realized that he still didn't want to tell everyone just yet, so he would start by bringing some gluten-free beer and eating before he went to the game. With these interim measures in place, as time passed, Mike felt stronger and more confident.

One night he surprised himself. When his friends were passing around the pretzels and Mike passed on them, he effortlessly mentioned why. In a few simple sentences that we had practiced, he told his buddies that he had been diagnosed with celiac disease, that some of the symptoms were bathroom trips, and that he couldn't eat the hoagies or drink the beer because they contained wheat and barley, which contain gluten.

Mike had some ready-made suggestions of gluten-free take-out places from his local celiac support group, and the poker group made a plan to pick up their refreshments from one of those places before the next poker night. It was all so easy. It didn't seem like a burden to his friends at all; they simply accepted it. The teasing also stopped.

All it took was for Mike to identify Dave as his ally and safe person; that eventually gave him the courage to tell the others.

identifying a friend
as a safe person

I bet you have one safe person in your life already. You may not have thought about him or her that way, but now that we've planted the conceptual seed, someone will probably pop up right away and make himself or herself known to you. Take a moment to think through the people in your life.

A safe person can be a family member, your romantic partner, or your best friend (and yes, you can have more than one). Start here: think of the word *safe*. Does one person automatically pop into your head? Go with your gut on this one. Don't second-guess or rationalize who you think it "should" be. What person, when you say the word *safe* to yourself, floats in front of your eyes? It's usually someone with whom you feel a close connection, a bond. Safe people are emotionally available and nonjudgmental, have an abundance of compassion, and are great listeners.

Once you've identified your safe person, let him or her know that you are dealing with some new feelings and that you could use some assistance (and in what ways). My friend Christopher and I have known each other since social work graduate school. I identified him as a safe person because our talks were always open, friendly, supportive, and loving. We have similar views of the world and a similar understanding of the importance of support, both as social work professionals and in our personal lives. Here's an example of what a phone conversation about being a safe person sounded like with Christopher: "Hey, Chris, sometimes I feel overwhelmed about having food allergies. I could really use some extra support, some extra-special Christopher-love. Can I call on you if I need to? Your friendship means so much to me, I'd appreciate your help. And of course, if you need anything from me, I'm there for you, too."

What friend could say no to that? After that conversation, Chris and I met for coffee and discussed some of the feelings I was having and how he could help. Dining out was a major stress, especially around our graduate school campus, where the food was fast and cheap but far from safe. Also, as a student government member, I attended work lunches with the faculty. When the president was involved, I felt extra intimidated. Chris listened intently, and we role-played some scenarios in which I told the president's secretary what I needed for work lunch. Chris and I plotted out some safer lunch places around the university, and I resolved to carry more snacks with me to be really safe. Practicing with Chris was a low-pressure situation, so we were able to try out all different kinds of conversations, which increased my confidence.

role-playing

Role-playing is a therapeutic or coaching tool in which you create a trial dialogue and act it out. You need two people to play. Each person takes an imaginary role and, in that role, plays out how a conversation might proceed. It's a very effective device for practicing how you want to say something, especially if you are imparting vital information and anticipate some resistance.

identifying a safe person
spontaneously

Sometimes (actually, most times) I still feel anxious about dining somewhere new, especially if the conversation with the restaurant management seems to be going downhill. (See chapter 11 for how to salvage a bad situation.) Having a safe friend with you can be invaluable, but you can also create one on the spot.

Danielle and I shared the same wonderful voice and performance teacher, Peggy. In that class, physical and emotional safety (only positive critiques and comments were allowed) was the number one priority, so you could perform and feel free to try out new attacks to a song. One night I was out with Danielle at a new, untested restaurant that had a very fishy and nutty menu, so I turned to my singing friend for some support. I told her what I was feeling and what I needed in order to feel better. She harbored no judgments, just a desire to help. It was lovely. Following is an example of how our conversation transpired. Notice how direct the conversation is, how simple it seems on the surface. But don't underestimate the simplicity; it takes practice to be this direct, vulnerable, trusting, and confident.

"I have to say," I began, "looking at the menu, I'm feeling a little nervous about dining here. It's all nutty salads or fish with nuts."

"What can I do? Do you want to go and try somewhere else?" Danielle asked.

"That's so sweet, thank you for the offer. Let's stay here and see what the manager says about how the kitchen can handle my allergies. I just wanted to give you a heads-up that I was feeling unsure about this menu."

"Of course. Whatever you need. Just let me know."

Isn't Danielle lovely? She was such a safe friend—what a relief. It was an on-the-spot I-need-some-help dialogue. Even though I hadn't identified Danielle as an official safe person, she certainly is one now. Most friends will be right there with you when you let them know what you need. Try it.

creating a safe person

If you think you don't have a friend who can be your safe person, you can create a safe person. Let's examine how I helped a food-allergy client create his safe person. As you read his story, try to think of someone in your life who might be like this.

Ben is a graduate student who's allergic to tree nuts. He attended a Worry-Free Dinners event, and after the dinner he realized that he could use some extra support to develop specific strategies to talk with friends, roommates, and romantic partners about his food allergies. He hired me as his food-allergy coach, and during the course of our treatment he told me the following story, which illustrates how a safe person functions:

> I was a little startled when my best friend Nikki swatted the bread stick out of my hand during dinner out one night and motioned for the server. "Are these bread sticks safe for my friend to eat?" Our server explained that after I told her I had a tree nut allergy, she had double-checked everything we'd ordered, and had included the breadsticks in her investigation with the chef. I had taken it for granted that our server would not serve us something potentially nut-contaminated but I hadn't asked about the breadbasket, an often overlooked nut situation. Nikki didn't overlook it, though. She thanked our server for being so meticulous, and explained that it would ease our dining experience if she would confirm the safety of the dishes. Nikki anticipated a potentially fraught situation and created a supportive environment for me to acknowledge my potential misstep, and also recover and investigate it myself. I snapped up a bite of the breadstick, feeling safe with my safe person.

Through our work together, Ben realized that Nikki was a perfect candidate to take on this level of friendship. Feeling more confident overall allowed him to identify his needs to Nikki, who took the extra step to support her friend with food allergies.

The beauty of the safe person is that whether you identify someone in your life who is already there or you create a safe person from a new friend, having that one person whom you can call on day or night, who won't judge you, and who will support you can help you to move forward with confidence. You need only one person completely in your corner. (If you have five, that's great, too.)

In both your inner circle and your outer circle of friends, there will be those who accept every aspect of you unquestioningly, those who will need your patience and some further education about your food-allergy diagnosis, and those who will be insensitive about this aspect of your life. Unlike your family (which you don't choose), your friendships are completely by choice and in your control.

understanding friends

Some friends show up on your doorstep with a compassionate, sympathetic, understanding quality already built in. They are naturally supportive, helpful, nonjudgmental, and accepting. Hold on to this type of friends; they are jewels.

Following are a few examples of the types of friends who seem to get it right away. I could tell by the language they used that they were supportive and kind people, that it would be easy to socialize with them, and that they didn't harbor judgments about food allergies or my medical requirements. Bonus: Be the friend you want to have in the world. If you want accepting, open, loving, and supportive friends, make sure that you are that kind of friend to others.

"You Pick"

I met Steve when I was studying abroad my senior year at Oxford University. We both belonged to the Oxford Star Trek Society, affectionately known as Trek Soc. We struck up a fast and easy friendship, because we both liked science fiction, Humphrey Bogart films, and eating. Steve knew that I had food allergies and asthma, but he didn't know the specifics.

The first time we went out for dinner, he said, "You pick the place. I'll eat anything, especially if it's fried." Steve immediately made the dining out process much easier. I suggested an English national pizza chain, which had a franchise in town. This began an ongoing weekly dinner date: we'd go and share an order of leek pizza to commemorate St. David, the patron saint of Wales (Steve is Welsh) and garlic dough balls, to commemorate the patron saint of all things garlic.

Once Steve asked if he could order a pizza with pine nuts. We wouldn't share it, obviously, but would it be okay if it were on the table, he wanted to know. If not, he'd order something else. He asked in such an open and honest way, just from a desire to know what to do and what I needed to stay safe. I knew there was a reason we liked each other immediately.

I said, "Eat whatever you like; just don't fling it on me." I was teasing, of course. (Humor, if you have it in your arsenal, is always helpful. Use it often.) This was a natural opportunity to give him a detailed five-sentence explanation of my food allergy situation so he would have a more nuanced understanding of my needs for future dining experiences.

"I'm allergic to tree nuts and salmon. Allergic reactions range from hives to wheezing to throat closing. I have medications on me at all times. It shouldn't be an issue, but if it is, I take the medication and we make a quick trip to the hospital. This is also why I can't try those mince tarts your mother sends from home; they're made with nuts."

Steve said, "Okay, got it. Let me know how I can help."

It was just that easy. It was a nonissue; it was effortless. It still is. We still dine together when he's in town—with an addendum: about ten years ago, Steve discovered that he's highly allergic to fish through an allergy incident while dining out. So now, when he and his nonallergic wife, Jemma, and their adorable nonallergic son, Dylan, visit and we all dine together, we both have the food-allergy talk with the server (see chapter 11), and we both carry autoinjectors of epinephrine and Benadryl.

"We Support You"

I was at a partly social, partly work dinner with new friends and work colleagues—a potential double whammy, in terms of social anxiety. I was with Francine, the editor in chief of an online food industry magazine, and Shari, a restaurant publicist who worked with the restaurant at which we were eating. The owner came by and chatted with Francine and Shari, giving me a perfect opportunity to have a conversation about my allergies.

Everything was going great, until the food arrived. The server was balancing a dish of bay scallops in sauce and my chicken au jus on the same arm. The scallop dish tipped a little, and some of the scallop sauce spilled onto the plate of chicken. We all watched it happen. The server put the food before me and began to walk away.

"I'm sorry, but I can't eat that," I said.

"It's just a little sauce," he said.

"As I mentioned, I'm allergic to salmon. I avoid all fish and shellfish, so I can't eat that chicken now because it has scallop sauce in it."

He took the plate back and brought it out a moment later. It was the same chicken with the sauce removed. By now, everyone at the table had their eyes on me as they waited to eat until this was sorted out. We were all going to have to wait a bit longer.

"I apologize for not being clearer," I said to the server, staying calm. "I need a whole different dish; this chicken was contaminated by the scallop sauce."

The server was now visibly annoyed. "Well, we'll have to start from scratch, you know. It'll take a while."

I had that split second of: What to do now? I wasn't going to eat the contaminated chicken, but everyone was waiting, their food getting cold. And these were new friends—what an introduction. Shari was sitting closest to me. She leaned over and said, "Do what you need to do. We support you." I asked the server to bring me a new chicken dish while everyone else started their food.

My chicken came out ten minutes later, and it was delicious. Shari, who was speaking for the group, made it clear that there was no judgment about my food allergies; everyone understood the implications and only wanted me to be safe. I felt such a wave of affection for my new friends. This was going to be so much easier because of her two sentences. Shari identified herself as a safe work friend. Listen for language like hers in the people around you.

The Food-Allergy Deputy

Some friends take it to the next level: not merely supporting you immediately, but advocating on your behalf. Sparkly jewels these are. This perfectly describes Vivi, my dear friend from college who became part of my inner circle of friends almost instantly. Vivi is a natural leader: warm, strong, incredibly capable, and outspoken in advocating for others.

In college, when we dined with a large group, I felt shy about shouting my allergy needs across a crowded table. (I still hate that; see chapter 11 for how to cope.) Vivi could see that I was struggling, so she would call the server over and prompt me with a gentle "Sloane, would you like to say something to the server before he leaves?"

When I was feeling shut out, Vivi opened a door. I get chills now just thinking about it. Food-allergy deputies are an excellent addition to your support system to help you ensure your food-allergy safety.

The Food-Allergy Bulldog

An offshoot of the food-allergy deputy is the friend (or family member or intimate partner) who wants to help so much that

be your own advocate

Whether you have one safe friend or one thousand safe
friends, you are the sheriff of Food Allergy Town. A deputy,
an ally, or an advocate should aid in ensuring that you get
what you need. If someone steps in and offers to speak
for you all the time, that's nice, but ultimately it's not really
helpful. You want support, not coddling, and it's a fine line.
You may need some coddling at some points until you feel
confident enough. We all need to take baby steps. Just
beware of allowing yourself to become complacent, relying
on anyone else for your safety. Your safety is always your job.

instead of receiving waves of love from him or her, you feel waves
of pressure. I've heard this time and again from food-allergy
coaching clients, and it's also happened to me. Some friends
bend over backward to accommodate you, which is a lovely trait,
but the attention becomes too much about your food-allergy
needs, your allergies, your possible deathly reactions, and your
medications.

Sometimes it's just too much you, you, you. "Where do you
want to go? Where do you want to eat? What about those? Can
you eat that, or that? What about this place? You pick the place?
Tell me what you want!" Sometimes you don't want all of this
attention. It can be exhausting to be the one choosing for everyone, all of the time.

Guilt inevitably sets in. Your friends want to help, and you want
them to help, but how do you get that to happen smoothly? A
variant of this occurs when your safe friend or inner-circle buddy
becomes a bulldog on your behalf, barking order to others at the
dinner table about your needs. All of a sudden there's a white-hot
spotlight on you again, even though it's all positive and good in
intention. Too much of this kind of attention can feel like social

pressure. There's a fine line between a safe friend and a "too much, too much" friend.

You don't want to be inconsiderate to the very people who want to support you, but getting everyone to calm down is another issue. Try saying a version of this the next time a food-allergy deputy crosses the line to food-allergy bulldog: "Thank you for watching out for me and for being so considerate. It's helped me to feel more confident, so much so that I think I can take it from here. I may still need your help from time to time, but I'm cool for now." Then make certain that you are cool when you are socializing with others.

the food-allergy talk with friends

An initial conversation with new friends about your dietary needs is a must if you plan on dining with them at any point. Even if you try to limit activities with friends to noneating events, it's bound to come up eventually, so meet the challenge head-on. Keep your food-allergy talk brief but educational; give the salient points and then move on. If your friends have more questions, add more educational information about symptoms, medications, your feelings, or how people can help you in an emergency, depending on the situation.

I recommend keeping the discussion breezy and light at the beginning of a friendship; you don't want to overwhelm a new acquaintance. It's important for you to judge what's necessary and when. Here's a sample conversation: "Before we eat, I should mention that I have some food allergies. I'm allergic to all tree nuts and salmon. I have medication with me; it shouldn't be an issue, but if it is, everything I would need is right here. So, have you been watching *Shark Week*? I'm obsessed!"

Five easy sentences, and you've told your new friend about your food allergies, where your medications are, what your needs are, and how he or she can help you. You've also relayed that you are comfortable, confident, and clear about your food allergies. You don't need to linger on this one aspect of your life; hence, the *Shark Week* comment. It's straightforward and very doable. Try it with your next new friend. (For the dating variation of the food-allergy talk, see chapter 6.) Food allergies are not the focus of any friendship, merely part of who you are, and a great friendship involves the coming together of two whole people.

breathing room

Like some of the families we discussed, some friends will need extra assistance in adjusting to your food allergies and continuing to be the loving friends you want and need. Take, for example, my dear friend Eric, whom I've known for years. When I see him, he'll invariably say, in an offhanded, joking way, "I don't get all of your allergies; they give me a headache." Or "I could never date you; just going out to dinner with you is too confusing."

Have you heard comments like these from close friends? Did you feel hurt or confused? Did you even write off these friends as unsafe? Did you get angry or defensive? All of those feelings are valid, and, depending upon the situation, I can understand why you'd feel defensive or want to fight back. Here's the challenge: Can you take a step back and hear what else might be going on underneath those seeming jabs? I know Eric well, and I know he is a deeply devoted friend; I also know that what Eric is really telling me is that my food allergies are overwhelming for him to handle, that he wants to make sure I'm safe but feels overpowered by their complexity and severity.

You didn't hear that? It's there. I know this because Eric is the kind of man who expresses his feelings with humor. A lot of people do that. So listen more closely next time, because buried within a funny jab may be the kernel of truth on which you need to build.

Like some of the family members we discussed, most of your friends will need some time to understand this part of you. Some may need a few dining excursions and to listen to you talk to the server; some will need to see how other friends handle it; and some will need just plain old time and patience.

In the meantime, take your food allergies off the friendship table. Food allergies are just one aspect of the totally great you, anyway. If a friend doesn't quite understand, that's okay. There are lots of other aspects of you to love and connect to. Give friends the space to get to know that part of you on their timeline; I bet they'll come around. (It may seem much harder, even impossible, to give family members or romantic partners space, but breathing room often works very well in those relationships, too.)

I used this tactic with Eric when he said those words to me. I gave him some breathing room and depersonalized. (Remember depersonalizing from chapter 4.) I smiled noncommittally and changed the topic. We continued to hang out, and sometimes even dine together with a group, but I made sure that food allergies weren't the topic of conversation.

Our friendship continued to grow and deepen, because food allergies were off the table for discussion I could enjoy all the other qualities about him: his humor, his loyalty, his honesty, and his support. In turn, because I wasn't self-righteous or angry at him for not getting it, he was able to connect to me in a deeper and more meaningful way. And what do you know? He came over one afternoon, walked into my kitchen to get a drink, and said, "I guess I should know more about these food allergies of yours. What can't you eat, again? Where's your medication? What do I need to do?"

With space and a nonjudgmental attitude from me, Eric came around in his own time. He's quickly become one of my fiercest supporters and advocates. Sometimes your friends just need some breathing room. Be generous; give them space to get to know this side of you.

teasing

There will be some friends in your life who will tease you about food allergies. They aren't the Erics of the world, or perhaps you've already tried the breathing-room technique and found out how un-Eric they are. This kind of teasing veers dangerously close toward hurtful. However, unlike extended family members, whom you might not see often or see only on holidays, one usually sees friends much more often, by choice. The technique that we explored in chapter 4 holds true for all interpersonal relationships, including friends and loved ones.

For example, do you have a friend who, every time you see each other, calls you "The girl [or guy] in a bubble"? Your first line of defense here is to depersonalize. Detach the comment from any negative feelings you have about your food-allergic life. Don't take the mean comment to heart. Take a breath and do not engage or respond. Ignore an insensitive statement; don't pay it any mind; just move on.

It's easier said than done, of course, and being able to detach from a mean comment often depends on the closeness of the friendship. If this is an outer-circle friend, someone you see rarely, or a friend of a friend, then it is probably not worth your time to engage this person. Let it go and move on. If this person wants to get to know you further, that's when it will be more appropriate to tell him or her how the comment makes you feel, because then the person will have the motivation to stop.

What if the person who's teasing you is someone closer, and you're having difficulty depersonalizing? Your next line of defense is the insensitive comment zigzag option that we explored in chapter 4. Acknowledge any truth in a joke, deflect the hurt, and move on to a different topic. You may feel like saying (or yelling), "Enough already with the same stupid food-allergy joke!" And you may end up saying that loud and often; however, it probably won't stop your friend from making this unfunny comment the next time he or she sees you.

Now that you have started doing all the work to accept this part of yourself—creating a Team You, talking with your family, identifying a safe friend—channel all of that support into your response. Be sweetness and light. Try saying a version of this, with a smile: "It's my happy bubble—join me! Hey, did you get a haircut? You look great!" The zigzag technique is to take the grain of truth (your world has to be more prescribed than most people's) and agree to it; deflect the mean part of the comment (you are different and should be separated from everyone else—so not true); and compliment the person as a way of moving on. When you don't respond to meanness with meanness, your friend will be disarmed and move on—usually.

What if a close friend constantly teases you, in public and in private, but you really like this person and want to continue the friendship? Here you may want to take a more direct approach, but this takes a lot of self-assurance. Practice first with a safe person (a family member, another friend, or an intimate partner), because this approach can be intense if you're not used to talking like this with your friends. When it's done well and with grace, however, it can bring friends closer.

Pull your friend aside quietly—in person is best (over the phone or in an e-mail can work, too, but beware of tone)—and say, "I know you love me, but when I'm called a "girl [or guy] in a bubble" it really hurts my feelings." Express your feelings and leave the conversation open-ended so your friend can respond. Use an "I" rather than a "you" statement ("I feel hurt" rather than "You hurt me"). "I" statements are excellent tools for being heard. Using "I" means that you're taking responsibility for your reactions and feelings. It's less threatening, and your friend will most likely be able to hear you and respond. The direct approach can feel like a confrontation or an attack when you start a sentence by saying "You," because it is. Consequently, when you start a direct discussion with "I," it's more of an invitation to begin a dialogue, not a litany of all the ways your friend has hurt you. Opening up a dialogue is your target with the direct approach. Try it; you will be rewarded.

If you've laughed off the comment and your friend persists in being insensitive, and you've had a direct "I"-statement dialogue and the friend still persists in being insensitive, then it's time to take a hard look at what else is going on in the relationship. Are there other problems or issues? Is your friend going through a difficult personal situation and acting out? Are there any other gaps in compassion for each other? Have there been similar break-downs of communication before? Is there an absence of mutual appreciation, kindness, or affection? Do your best to put aside your hurt feelings about mean statements and explore with your friend what's going on. Work toward reconnecting and reinvigorating empathy and compassion. Once those elements of your friendship are back in place, the teasing will die down and new bonds will be formed.

Friendship is truly a gift. Let your friends in on the food-allergic aspect of your life. Let them support you in ways you didn't even know you needed; in turn, support and accept them in ways you didn't even know you could. Remember that the deeper the communication is, the more satisfying the connection will be.

allergic girl's love letters

- Friendship is a rare gift; treasure the good friends you have by being the friend you would want.
- Friends come in all shapes, sizes, depths, and needs. At minimum, you need one ally, or advocate, in your friendship circle, one person who gets this aspect of you.
- Beware of allowing yourself to become complacent, relying on anyone else for your safety. Your safety is always your job.
- Most of your friends will understand your medical needs and accept that part of you.
- Some friends won't get the food-allergy thing immediately (or ever). Don't take it personally; there's still a lot to love, and they may get on board eventually.

- Some friends may tease you and not realize it's hurtful. There are many tools at your disposal for letting them know how you feel.
- If you need more support, turn to a food-allergy coach, family members, romantic partners, support groups, and online forums. Reach out—you are not alone.

6

your kiss is
on my list

Because your kiss is on my list
of the best things in life.
—Hall & Oates, "Kiss on My List"

The setting is an upscale restaurant in the Flatiron District of New York City at night. A man and a woman, their shoulders touching, seat themselves at the bar. Allergic Girl has soft brown curls and bright blue eyes. Cute Boy has affectionate green eyes and a shy smile. The din of a Saturday night quiets as the couple looks at the menu.

BARTENDER
What can I get you?

ALLERGIC GIRL
Hi. I have some food allergies I'd like to tell you about before we order.

BARTENDER

Sure. I'll get a pen to write these down. *(He reaches in his waistcoat for a pad and a pen.)*

ALLERGIC GIRL

Great. I'm allergic to *(she turns her head slightly so her date can hear)* all tree nuts, fish, and shellfish.

BARTENDER

(He takes down all of her requests, registering only a hospitable attitude.) OK, I'll let the kitchen know. We deal with these requests all the time. It will not be an issue.

ALLERGIC GIRL

Super! Thank you so much. *(Cute Boy has been poring over the menu; he seems very absorbed.)*

ALLERGIC GIRL

(Stroking the menu, running her light pink manicured nail over the entrée options.) Everything here is really delicious. So, what are you thinking of ordering?

CUTE BOY

(Extending his index finger) I think I'll have the halibut.

Allergic Girl reacts with disbelief; her jaw slackens and her eyes widen. Cute Boy doesn't notice as he's still looking at menu.

Cue the song "Kiss on My List" by Hall & Oates as Allergic Girl remembers past dates.

Allergic Girl is walking down the street hand-in-hand with date number two past the Plaza Hotel. Date number two stops to get hot sweet pecans from the roasted nuts vendor. Allergic Girl's face registers comical abject horror.

Allergic Girl and date number three are having a heated discussion with lots of hand motions. Date number three gestures down to the table. He seems to be saying something about "only a little bit" and holding Allergic Girl's shoulders, trying to lean in for a kiss. She backs away, insistently shaking her head. A look of extreme frustration crosses date number three's face. On their uncleared table are remnants of lamb chop bones on her plate and the skeleton of a salmon on his.

Allergic Girl is at a cozy New York City apartment house party. Date number four is eating smoked salmon salad out of Allergic Girl's sight. He puts his plate away, joins Allergic Girl, and kisses her on the neck. A huge hive welt forms where he's kissed her. She absentmindedly scratches her neck.

Allergic Girl and date number five are huddled in a cozy leather booth of a hotel bar. He's watching her intently as she points to the silver bowl of mixed nuts on the table. She gestures that she cannot have any or she will be very ill. Date number five calls over a server in a white coat, points to the dish and explains. The server removes the mixed nuts and brings some safe olives. Allergic Girl smiles widely and kisses date number five romantically. They settle into the booth for some serious canoodling.

Back at the upscale restaurant in the Flatiron District.

ALLERGIC GIRL
    If you eat the halibut (*beat*) I can't kiss you later.

CUTE BOY
    (*He does not look up from menu, does not move a muscle.
    He waits a double beat.*) I'll have the chicken.

We've all heard the expression "Be the star of your own movie," but dating and romantic relationships are the one place in which meet-ups feel like meet-cutes, conversations turn into snappy one-liners, situations take on screwball proportions, kisses can end in a mad dash to the pharmacy (think Will Smith in *Hitch*), and hookups can turn into a montage of embarrassments—all in a surreal cinemalike setting.

Are you the star with the key light? Or are you the quirky best friend? Maybe you're just a walk-on. Not good enough; it's time for you to get into romantic comedy. Getting into your "movie" when you have food allergies means taking control of your health and staying safe. Admittedly, taking control during the free fall of pheromones known as dating takes finesse. My advice is to let your dates in on this aspect of yourself just as you would with any new friend.

Like extended family and friends, romantic dates and long-term partners often fall into three categories in terms of understanding and accommodating your food-allergy diagnosis. There will be those who get it right away and are superflexible and accommodating. Most dates will need further education, explanations, and time to adjust. And there will be a few dates, and even some long-term romantic partners, who don't really understand your needs or what you're going through.

having "the talk"

Go back to your medical Team You, or follow up with reliable online resources for a refresher course on food allergies to assist you in explaining your needs with a date or romantic partner.

- American Academy of Allergy Asthma and Immunology (AAAAI.org)
- American College of Allergy, Asthma and Immunology (AACAAI.org)
- Anaphylaxis Canada (Anaphylaxis.ca)
- Asthma and Allergy Foundation of America (AAFA.org)
- Food Allergy Anaphylaxis Network (Foodallergy.org)
- Food Allergy Initiative (FAIUSA.org)

As we've seen with both family and friends, everyone around you—especially someone with whom you plan to be intimate—is going to need some food-allergy education. That's why it's imperative for you to have the answers. How, when, and where you impart that education is up to you, and there are myriad ways to get it done. Keep your intention clear: in dating, the goal is to get to know another person and to let him or her get to know you. Food allergies are part of you. At some point, you'll want to let this person know that part of you.

everyone has something

Unlike your family or even your friends, dating involves a whole set of extra variables that seem to obfuscate the interaction. I say *seem to* because your feelings, thoughts, and attitudes about a medical diagnosis can often do more injury to a potential relationship than the medical diagnosis itself. So if you've gotten this far in the book and you're still feeling self-conscious about having adverse reactions to food when you meet new people, know this: *everyone has something.*

Think about it another way. Which friends, work colleagues, and friendly acquaintances don't complain about some aspect of their lives? Whether it's weight gain or weight loss, money troubles or in-law troubles, hairlines that recede or hair that grows in unwanted locations, lack of sleep or chronic oversleeping, a doughnut problem or a video game problem, everyone has something.

It's what makes us unique. Embrace this aspect of your uniqueness and embrace the uniqueness in those around you. Level the playing field right now. Disclose this part of yourself to a potential sexy-time partner. The immediate reward is an open and honest connection to another human being—even if it never goes past drinks.

the food-allergy talk

Food-allergy diagnoses are on the rise worldwide, and media outlets frequently report on food allergies. The odds are that a new
acquaintance will have heard or seen a news story. This will make
introducing the topic easier, but keep in mind that new people
in your world will not have the intimate knowledge they need
about your food allergies, and they certainly won't know about
your needs until you tell them. It's your job to clue in a potential
date about your food-allergic needs.

I call it the food-allergy talk. This is not a where-is-the-
relationship-going talk. Not at all. This is an I-need-to-tell-you-
something-about-me-so-we-can-have-the-best-time-ever talk. It's
purely informational. It's a medical fact about you. Remember, connect to your food-allergy needs without shame, embarrassment, or
apology; communicate those needs clearly, assertively, and graciously;
and recognize that you have options. When you are able to state this
about yourself with confidence, you will get that attitude echoed back
to you. For example, if your attitude is positive and light, your date
will probably take on that attitude as well. If your attitude is defensive
or unsure, your date may mirror that back to you, too. Keep that
information tucked away as you begin to have these talks with dates.

You can influence the outcome of the food-allergy talk with
dates. If you haven't done so already, go back and spend some
time working through your feelings about having food allergies.
Practice talking about your food allergies with supportive family
members or with your safe friend so you can develop an easy and
confident attitude. Role-play, using the suggested scenarios and
language described in the following sections.

When to Introduce the Food-Allergy Talk

Dating in New York City often involves dining out, so the
food-allergy talk comes up pretty darn fast, sometimes even
before the date transpires. For example, Sol and I met while we

were both dining alone at the bar of a restaurant. He overheard me talking to the bartender about my allergies, and he joined in the conversation.

The day before our first date, I received this e-mail from him: "What would you think of going to a restaurant in SoHo? I spoke with them, they're really nice, they have Mediterranean-influenced food with a big emphasis on using seasonal items, and they can definitely work with any allergy request." He had gone ahead and told the restaurant all my food-allergic needs (downloaded from my Allergicgirl.com blog), so the staff was prepared for me.

When we sat down to dine, I told Sol where my medications were, just in case, and reiterated my needs to the server and the manager. He was right; they were prepared for me. We shared allergen-free dishes, a total *Lady and the Tramp* scenario. Sol did all of the legwork so I could dine out safely; it was excellent.

Depending on your age, circumstance, interests, and geographical location, dining out together may not be at the top of your list of first-date activities. When you can, suggest non-food-related dates for the few first get-togethers. Drinks, parties, concerts, comedy clubs, walks, car rides, sports, beaches—there are plenty of places that don't involve sitting down and dining.

It's okay to delay the food-allergy talk until you get to know someone better. If you're feeling shy or uncertain (or have felt burned from past negative experiences), ease into it. Bonus: If you're having a nonfood date, don't go hungry. Eat before you go, and bring a safe snack in case you get hungry later. Have a plan: know of places near your date where you can grab safe food if you need to, and always have your medications on hand in case you end up dining out.

The Basics of the Food-Allergy Talk

Once you're ready to introduce the topic, or it comes up naturally in conversation, the basics of the food-allergy talk can be as elaborate or as simple as the situation demands. You will need to figure out what is appropriate and when; know that that will change with time, with the people, and with the scenario.

Work out a few versions that you're comfortable with for where you are right now. The basic components should include what food allergies are (the body's swift immune response to an offending food), what can happen from exposure (hives, itching, wheezing, anaphylaxis), what medication to use in an emergency (Benadryl, epinephrine, cortisone, an inhaler), where the medication is kept (your pocket, purse, book bag, briefcase), and how to use the medication (swallow, inhale, or jab).

Sometimes the talk is the simple truth: "If you eat that, I can't kiss you"—as I said to Cute Boy. Sometimes a more elaborate explanation is required. It's up to you, as long as you get it done. Your approach should be friendly; smile a lot and be your wonderful, lovable self. If you're naturally funny, use that; humor is a wonderful way to diffuse tension and impart information. This is serious, possibly life-saving stuff, but you're still on a date and having fun. Let your partner know that you accept this part of yourself by being confident about what you say and how you say it. Actress Carrie Fisher, in her one-woman show *Wishful Drinking*, said, "Say your weak thing in a strong voice." I'd add, say your weak thing in a funny voice, if you need to. When talking with your date, make eye contact but don't glare. Keep your face and your body language relaxed. Practice in a mirror or, better yet, with one of your safe friends or someone from your inner circle. Like a spoonful of sugar, humor helps the food-allergy talk go down much easier.

Come up with your versions in your voice but try these on for fit and feel:

- *Direct version:* "I have food allergies. If you want to kiss me as much as I want to kiss you, please don't eat any tree nuts or salmon. I'm really allergic to those and can't kiss you if you eat them."

- *Simple version:* "I should let you know that I have severe food allergies to tree nuts and salmon. I carry medication with me in my purse just in case; here it is. The odds are that nothing will happen, but I wanted to let you know."

- *Humorous version 1:* "You know that scene in *Pulp Fiction* when John Travolta stabs Uma Thurman in the heart with adrenaline? Well, I have one of those pens in case I have a severe food-allergic reaction. Just don't stab me in the heart; it goes into the thigh."

- *Humorous version 2:* "Remember that scene in *Hitch*, where Will Smith has an allergic reaction and his face blows up? That'll be me if you eat nuts or salmon and I kiss you."

- *Elaborate version:* "Just to give you a heads-up, I have some severe food allergies. I'm allergic to tree nuts and salmon. If I accidentally ingest them, I could get an itchy mouth or throat, my face or lips may swell, or I could get hives or start wheezing. If any of that happens, I have emergency medication right here in my purse. Here's the Benadryl; I should take two and possibly use the autoinjector of epinephrine: pop the cap and jab it into my thigh. My in-case-of-emergency numbers are in my phone under ICE. It is doubtful that any of this will happen, but I wanted you to know."

- *Bonus addition* (I said this to LT from the prologue and Dean in the scenario on the following page): "I might not realize that I'm having an allergic reaction. I might just look panicky, start clearing my throat, or complain of itchy ears. Hives may appear that I can't see. If you notice any of those symptoms, tell me, and I should take a Benadryl." In LT's case it was prescient: hives I couldn't see broke out everywhere, and I wasn't quick to take my Benadryl until he prompted me. I was thankful that he was so caring and listened so closely.

Now let's look at some of these food-allergy talks in action.

"what do i need to do?"

I met Dean at an food-industry event. He's a photographer and was hired to chronicle the event. I noticed him noticing me; he took my picture, and I asked for a copy (sly, I know). We exchanged cards and e-mails and then made a date. We attended another food-industry cocktail event, smooched, and then separated, because I had an invitation to a vegan fundraiser at an art studio and he had an invitation to a tourism board event that was showcasing shellfish.

Dean knew that I was a writer and a food-allergy coach, but he didn't think about how that might translate to an intimate situation. After an hour at our respective events, we re-met. As he approached to open my car door, he extolled the towers of shrimp, lobster, and other fishy delights he had just consumed. He then went in for a big wet "hello" kiss. I pulled back gently.

"Didn't you just eat fish?"

"Yes, it was great! Lobster, oysters, salmon . . . "

"I'm sorry, I can't kiss you. I'm allergic."

"Okay," he said, recovering quickly. "What do I need to do? Drink water? Gargle? Brush my teeth?"

I was so relieved. This is exactly the response I would want from a date. It was a response of someone who cared about my well-being and was clearly motivated to do what he had to do so I could stay safe. If Dean had said: "Can't I just kiss you anyway?" or "I only ate a little shellfish, c'mon, it can't hurt," the conversation would have been much different. Dean gave me the perfect lead-in to tell him about my food allergies and what we needed to do ensure that I was completely safe and could enjoy myself.

With time and experience, I've learned that a good date will never shame you about a medical need—once you make it clear that it's a medical need. It's part of who you are, and your date already likes you. A mark of a good date, or at least someone you can kiss and get to know better, is that he or she will want to know what to do in order to be with you.

I had recently reread the seminal study on peanut proteins in saliva—lucky me. So I had the answer for Dean's question at my fingertips. The *Journal of Allergy and Clinical Immunology* published a study in 2006 that concluded,

> With respect to advice regarding avoidance of kiss related reactions, the safest approach we advocate is for the partner of the individual with allergy to avoid the allergenic food. For peanut butter specifically, we have shown that interventions that include a waiting period and brushing teeth/chewing gum appear to reduce the concentration to levels that are unlikely to induce reactions, but did not reduce [the peanut protein] Ara h 1 to undetectable in all cases. Waiting several hours after peanut butter consumption and eating a meal within that time frame should reduce protein levels in saliva to clinically insignificant quantities. On the basis of our time course results from 30 participants, there is 95% confidence that levels of [the peanut protein] Ara h 1 in saliva will reach undetectable levels (<20 ng/mL) for 90% of people several hours after peanut butter consumption and after a meal.

Back to Dean. I said, as adorably as possible, "We need to wait a bit and eat a nonallergenic meal."

"Cool," Dean said, and off we went to grab a burger at a place that makes only burgers; no fish, no nuts. We talked more about what my food allergies were, where my medicines were kept in my purse, and what to do in case of an emergency. Dean listened intently and asked a few questions to confirm that he understood, and we kept eating. Midway through our allergy-safe dinner, he smiled and said, "May I kiss you now?" We had a big smooch-a-thon right there at the burger restaurant. Fishy crisis averted, and we had a great date.

It sounds supereasy, doesn't it? You can make it just that easy. It's within your power to make that happen. Communicating your needs clearly will invariably receive a clear response. I know this because it's Newton's third law of motion: Every action has an equal and opposite reaction. Communicate kindly and clearly, and you will receive a clear and kind communication in return. Dean asked me what he needed to do to be kissable; I said we needed to wait and he needed to eat something without that allergen. Bonus: I asked Dean recently what he thought about that whole exchange. He said he appreciated knowing what he needed to do. He added that someone who wouldn't want to know what to do "didn't deserve a kiss." I couldn't have said it better myself.

"is there anything i can do?"

Food-allergy coaching client Ben and I worked on how to talk with potential kissing partners to impart vital information in a way that was comfortable. Ben told me this recent kissing and food-allergy story in which he employed the strategies we had role-played:

> I tried to smack the chocolate out of Paul's hands, but Paul thought we were playing some sort of game and quickly popped it in his mouth. I needed to let my kissing buddy know that he just ate my most dreaded food-allergy adversary: the hazelnut. On a recent skin test at my allergist's office, the prick from hazelnut consumed all the other scratch-test bumps, taking most of my arm with it. As Paul sidled up to me on the dance floor, I edged carefully away.
>
> I took him outside the dance club to explain. "That chocolate contains hazelnuts. I can't kiss you now. Remember we talked about that earlier?" Paul looked

crestfallen. "But," he said, "I checked the packaging, there were no nuts listed!" I explained that sometimes labels for individually wrapped products, like chocolate or other candy, don't paint the whole picture; you have to look at the original box. "I'm so sorry, is there anything I can do?" So cute, so thoughtful and well meaning.

You [Sloane] had sent me the peanut study that demonstrates that the only thing to do is wait and eat something else. "Here, eat this apple." I quickly thrust the safe snack I had with me into his hand. Paul happily obliged. While he was eating, I described the study so Paul could have some background. Paul listened, eyes widening. "Okay, so let's wait a few hours to be safe," Paul said. I reached around to grab his hand, but he stopped me. "Just to be safe, let me wash my hands before you do that. I wouldn't want to hurt you."

Ben explained his needs clearly; he even used research to back up his point. His date understood not only what to do but also the seriousness of the situation, and he said the best date thing ever: "I wouldn't want to hurt you." Of course not. A good date, once he or she knows the situation, would never want to hurt you; he or she likes you and wants to be with you.

"my sixth sense"

Kyle Dine is a food-allergy educator, musician, and youth leader for Anaphylaxis Canada. He's severely allergic to peanuts, tree nuts, eggs, mustard, and penicillin and had this to say about food allergies, dating, and the food-allergy talk:

I've never been one to go out for dinner on a first date unless I am very comfortable with that person. I much prefer a coffee date so there doesn't have to be food involved. I have many food-ordering routines and would prefer to introduce my allergies gradually to a new date rather than right away in a restaurant setting. I do communicate my allergies and associated risks very early in the relationship, but usually once I feel that they have gotten to know the real me, with or without allergies. When it comes to how I tell them, I'm pretty frank, but consciously trying to make it sound not scary, but manageable.

For example, I once offered to lend a pen to a girl so she could write something down and pulled out my autoinjector, which stirred up a great laugh and opened the door for a conversation about my allergies and why I carry it. Another example: I list a few popular junk food things that I can't eat and say that you could view it as a highly disciplined diet. I do tell dates that my allergies are life threatening, but again, usually with humor—that is, my nut detection skills are my sixth sense; if you ever tried to kiss me after eating nuts, you would find my hand coming up between us as a reflex. Early on in a relationship I don't expect them to learn everything about food allergies, but if they have an open mind and are willing to help, it is a very good sign.

Kyle uses humor in way that makes him extra charming to a potential date. You can do that, too. The point here is that you are on a date. Get to know the person and let him or her get to know you. Find a natural opportunity and get in there and have the food-allergy talk.

Dating with food allergies can be relatively effortless, even with a medical diagnosis that requires some care from your potential partner. It can be drama-free. What's most crucial is that you know what to do in an emergency so that you do not rely on anyone other than yourself to keep you safe. When you're dating, becoming romantically involved, and eventually partnering up, it is great when that partner wishes to know more about how to help you, what to do, what to avoid, and how to nurture you. That is ideal, and it is what many of us look for in a partner. Dating is how you find out who people are, so get your date on and do it safely.

As with friends and family members, some dates or relationship partners will take longer to truly understand the ins and outs of food allergies and all of the components involved: not merely kissing or being intimate, but cooking for each other, dining together, and being together for other food-related activities. There are all kinds of variations. Most of the time it just takes some further explanation; rarely, is it a lost cause. Dating is about finding out.

"don't try to be a hero"

Kyle told me that some dates took a bit longer to understand his medical needs:

> A few ex-girlfriends might have been completely overwhelmed at first, as they had never met someone with severe food allergies. Their first connection is usually with the life-threatening part, and they don't consider that you can live safely with food allergies. I think the key to whether they get it or not is their openness to learn. If they won't put in the time to learn how to keep me safe, I wouldn't have time for that relationship.
>
> For example, when cooking I'm double-checking labels and also keeping kitchen surfaces clean. I am a clean-kitchen freak. I wouldn't be comfortable if a girlfriend left knives with peanut butter (one of my allergies) hanging around the sink or other shared areas. Most girlfriends did get it eventually, but one common issue was how much they got it, and how it would translate into a safe meal made by either them or their parents. There were a few meals where an ex either made

a slipup or didn't communicate all of my allergies to her parents, who made the meal. They were honest mistakes, and luckily I asked questions before the meals and found they weren't safe. I was much more involved in the cooking process afterward.

This alone changed how I date: letting girlfriends know that they don't have to try to be a hero by trying to prove they can make safe meals for me. I'm very honest in letting them know that cooking for me is no easy task. I usually cite a few alternate words for my allergens, which can be found (or missed) on food labels, such as *albumin* for egg and *marzipan* for almond paste. They usually understand at this point that a lot more goes on behind cooking a safe meal than simply looking for a "peanut-free" label or logo on a package of food. I really appreciate their effort, but ultimately I need to be involved in the process in order to have a comfortable meal.

Kyle demonstrates here that open communication is vital. Trust, another component, is built over time. Especially with someone who knows nothing about food allergies, the learning curve will be steep. Make sure to keep yourself as safe as Kyle did by asking questions, and not relying on secondhand information, until your new date or potential partner has gotten the hang of it. It may take you a lifetime to get it, so cut your dates some slack if they don't get it right away. And make sure you keep yourself safe.

"you think i don't know that?"

The above quote comes from comedian Martin Short, playing attorney Nathan Thurm on *Saturday Night Live* in the 1980s, and it sums up the attitude of the date I'm going to tell you about.

It's been a rare date who's made fun of me or shamed me in any way about food allergies. By rare, I mean once in recent history, that I can recall. Considering that I have had food allergies my entire life and have been dating for more than twenty years, those are fantastic odds. But because it did happen once, recently, it's worth sharing.

For many of you, this is one of your dating nightmares: a date who not only doesn't understand your food allergies but actually makes fun of you. If I had felt even the tiniest bit unsure, ashamed, or uneasy about having food allergies, being teased by a date would have been uncomfortable at best and humiliating at worst. However, after doing my best to communicate my needs to my date (and being rebuffed at every turn) I understood this date's reaction for what it was: more information about who he was and what a relationship with him might have been like.

As we lingered over our second drink, my just-drinks date with Adam turned into a let's-get-something-to-eat date. There was a place nearby, I remembered in my tipsy haze, that I had been to before. I knew the menu was simple, not overly nutty or fishy, and that if I ordered something straightforward I should be relatively safe. We got in line.

"So if I order something that you can't eat, could we still . . . er . . . I mean . . . what do I need to not eat in order that we could . . .?" Adam was asking me about kissing me and food allergies. We hadn't had the food-allergy talk yet, but he knew about my allergies because we had spent some time talking about what we do for a living. I zoomed through the food-allergy talk covering the important highlights: "I'm allergic to all tree nuts, fish and shellfish. They don't have fish or nuts here, so order whatever you like; it should be fine." It was a condensed version of the longer talk, but it would do in a pinch.

We kissed before the meal—a nice start. When we sat down with our respective orders and ate, I wondered: What if my calculations were wrong? What if there was something I was allergic to in this restaurant, in either his dish or mine, and we kissed again? What if something happened and Adam had no idea what to do? I decided to make a bold move and just give him my five-sentence run-down of the situation, since kissing was probably going to happen again.

"I should probably show you what to do if there's a food-allergy emergency, just in case."

I started by mentioning Benadryl, to which he rolled his eyes. "Don't you think I know what Benadryl is? Any idiot knows what that is."

I forged ahead, taking out the autoinjector of epinephrine just so he could see it, but Adam wasn't listening. He seemed very focused on making loud, inappropriate jokes—about me, about food allergies, and about Benadryl. Even the diners at the next table looked over with sympathetic glances. It was obvious: this date was tumbling downhill, and fast. We had spent the earlier part of the evening trying to find common ground, without succeeding, and now this.

Clearly, Adam was nervous, and making jokes was making him feel better. But it wasn't making me feel that good. What tiny potential there may have been evaporated. We said good night quickly after that, and even though he e-mailed me for another date, I declined. Ultimately, we hadn't connected on any level, and the joking was the last nail in the proverbial date coffin.

long-term relationships

Once you've dated and gotten to know someone and become exclusive, you enter relationship-land. Intimate relationships require more negotiation and honest communication and are founded upon deeper feelings of trust. Kyle told me how he and his fiancée have worked out some of the finer details:

> I am rather lucky in the fact that my fiancée has celiac disease. Although we have been together for a number

of years, we continually find ourselves having to adapt to new risks and situations together. The keys for us have been solid communication of our comfort levels, as well as a willingness to compromise. We have adopted each other's allergies, in a way, but not completely. I have made the switch to gluten-free pizza and pasta, and she has switched from many of her usual brands to ones that are allergy-friendly for me.

I think the biggest benefit of having a fiancée who does get it is support. Difficult social situations have only gotten easier, because I know she's got my back, whether it's asking about ingredients or educating others about allergies.

Support is one of the best things about a long-term relationship, and Kyle and his fiancée sound like they do a great job of supporting each other.

Most of my clients in long-term relationships have partners who are incredibly supportive about their food allergies. My experiences have mostly mirrored that empirical data: long-term partners generally get it and do what they can to support this part of you. For example, when I asked my ex-boyfriend Henry recently about how he dealt with my food allergies, he said that three days before seeing me he would stop eating tree nuts and fish—just to be on the safe side. He did this of his own accord; I had no idea. I had been very open with him about my food allergies, and he took it upon himself to eliminate that concern from our intimate relationship. It was that straightforward.

missteps and miscommunications

Often, what partners may not fully comprehend is the deep and lasting anxiety or even trauma associated with having food allergies and the prospect of a food-allergic reaction. Here's a typical example from an Allergicgirl.com blog reader:

> I was in my early 20s, in New England with my boyfriend at the time. Even though he knew I'm allergic to all seafood, he insisted on taking me to a seafood restaurant. I didn't want to make a scene, so I ordered plain pasta. But in my mind, I couldn't stop imagining that they were cooking my pasta in the lobster pot cooking water. I wanted to leave; my boyfriend thought I was crazy and wouldn't budge. I left in tears, and—needless to say—broke up with him shortly thereafter. He so didn't get it.

Whatever's going on in your head can really do a relationship in, especially if your partner doesn't understand, accept, or support this part of you.

There's been only one long-term relationship that I can recall in which we got into an argument about food allergies, about what I would or wouldn't eat. On a deeper level, the argument was not about food allergies at all, but about compassion and a perceived lack of understanding. Add to that several other problems in the relationship, and this incident was merely one example of some of the deeper issues that would eventually break up the relationship.

The argument was during our second year together. Rick had moved to Los Angeles for work, and we were trying to maintain a long-distance relationship. It wasn't working. What had been gaps in communication turned into chasms. There were phone fights and texted apologies; missed connections and hurt feelings. I flew out for one final visit, and that was the last time we were together. Rick took me to a very well-known Los Angeles restaurant for dinner. He had been there many times and really wanted me to try its famous bread, which arrives at your table right out of the oven. I asked our server what was in the bread.

"It's a secret recipe. I can't tell you," he said.

"But I have food allergies. I can't eat it without knowing what's in it."

"Sorry, ma'am. It's a secret family recipe, and I can't divulge its ingredients. If you tell me what you're allergic to, I can tell you if it's in there."

"Well, tree nuts to start."

"There are no tree nuts in the bread." And off he walked. Of course, that wasn't going to be good enough. This is when Rick became surprisingly insistent.

"He said it had no nuts. Try it. It's really so good, I know you're going to love it."

"Thanks, but I can't. I don't know what's in it."

A power play ensued: Eat it. No, I can't eat it. The back-and-forth became heated. After two years, Rick still didn't understand

Couples Counseling

Do you need assistance in your relationship? Couples counseling, whether for short-term or long-term spans, can be highly beneficial. Here are ways to find a reputable couples counselor.

- Ask your managed care provider or health care insurer for names.
- Go back and read chapter 2 on how to get a good referral from friends.
- Find a social worker (someone with an MSW) from the National Association of Social Workers, www.socialworkers.org.
- Find a psychologist (PhD) through the American Psychological Association, www.apa.org.
- Find a psychiatrist (MD) through the American Psychiatric Association, www.psych.org.
- Find a mental health professional through the National Institute of Mental Health, www.nimh.nih.gov/index.shtml.

that if I didn't know what was in something, I couldn't eat it. We tried to continue the dinner in a pleasant way, but his frustration was palpable, and my reaction to his frustration was even more so.

When we got back to Rick's apartment, we talked it through. He said he "felt sorry for" me. I was hoping for some compassion, understanding, and consideration; the last thing I wanted from my romantic partner was pity. Pity has no place in a loving, mature relationship, which, it was becoming all too clear, Rick and I didn't have. (I get a little defensive thinking about it, even now, years later.) With Rick, my restricted diet pushed other relationship concerns to the forefront, and this visit was the beginning of the end.

A lack of understanding about food allergies is not a good enough reason to break up with a long-term partner, but a lack of understanding, compassion, emotional support, and accommodation of a medical need is another matter. This lack may indicate that there are larger issues in the relationship. These issues should be examined and discussed thoroughly before any conclusion is made. Very often, when the underlying issues are resolved, your food allergies become what they should be: fully accepted and a nonissue.

Dating can be allergy-free and drama-free. Long-term relationships built on trust, love, and open communication can be beautifully supportive, often in ways you couldn't have anticipated. Acceptance of your food allergies as an aspect of who you are helps your partners to get on board. When a date or a partner doesn't understand your food needs right away, don't get defensive, get investigative: try exploring what's going on, without drama, to uncover how to proceed. Whether you're on a date or in a long-term committed relationship, how you handle your medical diagnosis and how your date or partner handles it is just more information about you, the other person, and your (possibly) fantastic food-allergy-free couplehood.

allergic girl's kissing list

- Dating is about getting to know someone and letting that person get to know you, food allergies included.
- Level the dating playing field by recognizing that *everyone has something*.
- Tell dates about your food allergies, either right away or later, but get it done. Give them time and space to get on board.
- Most dates want to know this about you; they want to know what to do in an emergency and how they can help (and not hurt you in any way).
- It's a rare date who will shame you. If a date does, treat it as more information about that person and how you two might interact on other levels.
- A long-term partner can be your safe person, providing compassion, understanding, support, and trust.
- If food allergies create tension in your dating or long-term relationship, look at what else is going on. Work toward building on the positives and creating an environment of support.
- For more support within a long-term romantic relationship that isn't working, seek out couples counseling or food-allergy coaching.

7

life's a banquet

I've come for my weekly shopping trip at Fairway Market on the Upper West Side of Manhattan, and I'm armed. The aisles are narrow and cramped; there are always hordes of people, and everyone's feisty. It's part of the charm. Don't come to Fairway unless you're ready to do battle. Every shopper has a personal battle-ready routine.

I'm a strategic shopper: I have a list, I know what I need, and I go right to it. Some days I shop with an eye to try something new, so I let my eye wander to a new brand of a trusted item: Lebanese yogurt instead of Greek yogurt, or blood oranges from Italy instead of navel oranges from Florida. I allow time for accidental wanderings into aisles rarely visited or products previously over-looked, but mainly I have my mission and my list. I head straight for the produce, right inside the main door.

Salad greens and carrots are the first two items in my basket. Then I start *recipizing*. Is that asparagus on sale? I could roast it with olive oil and a squeeze of lemon juice as a side dish; if it's really cheap, maybe I'll make a soup as well. The heads of radic-chio look robust. Is that fresh fennel down the aisle? And are those oranges on sale—four for three dollars? A radicchio, fennel, and orange salad with an orange vinaigrette would be heavenly.

Keep your diet varied, mostly plants and mostly unprocessed, is what Michael Pollan says in *The Omnivore's Dilemma*. So salad, yes. But maybe some French feta cheese (it's milder than Greek feta), with French niçoise olives—they're perfectly piquant. Roasted beets in olive oil and sea salt are very simple and deli-cious. Some red chard, sautéed with garlic, ginger, and some of those blood oranges, with orange zest, might also be delicious.

Fairway is a place to savor all of the goodies around you. At the end of the salad aisle, by the towers of mushrooms, I dash past the milk, yogurt, and butter, past the prepared-foods coun-ter to the chickens roasting on a spit all the way in the back. (A Fairway shopping secret: if you go around eleven o'clock at night, the chickens are two for one and the lines are almost non-existent.) The roasted, kosher, and free-range chickens have no spices, no fillers, and no extras. I pick one that looks like it hasn't completely surrendered to the rigors of roasting and head to the next large room, slinking past my fellow shoppers in the cash-only line and up the side stairs, to the organics section. Upstairs is not only the organic produce but also aisles upon aisles of gluten-free, allergen-friendly packaged goods. The mundane nature of food shopping is enlivened by so many possibilities. Knowing that I'll have a full fridge and pantry, that I'm able to feed myself safely and well, is a source of personal pride. In the case of someone with

allergic girl's favorite shopping spots in new york city

- Bell Bates: http://bellbates.com for herbs and spices
- Fairway Market: www.fairwaymarket.com
- Farmers' markets: www.grownyc.org/greenmarket for locations
- Han Ah Reum Mart: www.hmart.com/ for Korean foods and ingredients
- Kalustyan's: www.kalustyans.com/ for Indian foods, herbs, and spices
- Pearl River Mart: pearlriver.com for Chinese foods and nonperishables
- Westerly Natural Market: www.westerlynaturalmarket.com
- Whole Foods: www.wholefoodsmarket.com

food allergies (that is, a restricted diet), so much depends on a full fridge with safe-for-you-foods.

the foodie in every food-allergic person

I admit it: I'm a total foodie. You are, too.

Read this definition of *foodie* from Wikipedia: "Foodies love food for consumption, study, preparation, and news. . . . Foodies want to learn everything about food, both the best and the ordinary, and about the science, industry, and personalities surrounding food" (http://en.wikipedia.org/wiki/Foodie).

You fit the criteria. As someone with food allergies, by necessity, you have to pay deep and almost obsessive attention to everything you consume in order to stay reaction-free and safe. You study ingredients and labels. You ask about food preparation and presentation, whether in a restaurant or at your Aunt Bea's house. You read news articles about new foods for the food-allergic community and foods that have been tainted and may not be appropriate for you. You explore what's right for your diet and what you need to eliminate. So, according to the Wikipedia definition, people with food allergies are foodies by virtue of their intense relationship to food.

Do you still think that having allergies is not foodie fabulous but a downer, even a burden? That the constant reading of labels and asking questions of servers, chefs, caterers—everyone—a drag? Does the self-consciousness that comes with having food allergies still have a small sting?

Know this: everyone has a relationship to food. It may be positive or it may be negative; people may not realize that they think about it, but even the absence of a relationship is a relationship. Some of my happiest memories are of food, and some of my scariest life moments have involved consuming an ingredient to which I reacted badly. I bet you have similar feelings, a need to reconcile these two disparate feelings. My relationship to food could have remained negative, traumatized, and distrustful, but instead it's transformed into something joyful, pleasurable, and gratifying.

How did I reconcile those two disparate experiences? How does anyone? I was able to do it because I recognized that there's an inner foodie, or food lover, in me. I know there's one in every food-allergic person, and that includes you.

It's commonly believed that noted psychoanalyst Carl Jung said, "In the symptom is the symbolic solution." For those of us with adverse reactions to food, who, because of those reactions feel like we hate food, the solution may be to embrace food, to love food. Think of it this way. Elie Wiesel, the noted author and humanitarian, is quoted as saying: "The opposite of love is not hate, it's indifference." So if you hate what food can do to you, that means you also have the capacity to love what food can do for you. I don't think any of you are indifferent to food and its effects on your body and your psyche, just the opposite: you are passionate about food because you need to be. The challenge is to reframe your food relationship from one that may feel negative to one that feels more positive.

where you are right now

If you're at the beginning of your food-allergy-diagnosis acceptance process, still sorting out the scary feelings after a particularly severe reaction or after receiving the diagnosis, then it's definitely enough to just deal with where you are right now. You may be feeling antifood or think that allergens are the enemy. Feel your feelings, even when they're uncomfortable. Start to track (make a mental or physical note) when you feel them: at family events, at work functions, with your loved ones, or all the time.

Teaching yourself to become aware of your feelings is vital. Listen to the voice in your head; what is it saying? You're scared, you're helpless, you're alone? These are all normal feelings. What will help you is to move through what we explored in the first two sections. If you haven't started working through those sections, start now; it will help you travel along the arc of your negative feelings toward acceptance.

Are you feeling scared? Acknowledge that food allergies and the possibility of a severe reaction is scary; it's undeniable. That is the reality. Are you feeling helpless? Find an allergist with whom you connect and trust. Discuss your diagnosis with a qualified medical professional, explore your concerns, and generate concrete goals (like an emergency plan of action and how and when to use medications). Seeing an allergist who supplies valid information for your needs will help you to feel less helpless while ensuring your safety in all circumstances. Are you feeling alone? Start having conversations about your feelings, thoughts, concerns, and even fears (rational or irrational—they are all valid) with your friends and family. Identify a safe friend, the one person on your side who will help you more than you know. (Go back to chapter 5 to find that safe friend.) Are you feeling stressed? De-stress by adding (or resuming) physical activity—the gym, biking, hiking—yoga, meditation, or deep breathing. If you're a talker, grab a safe friend and talk it out. If you're arty, express your feelings through arts or crafts. If you're a mover, go dance it out.

If you are actively working on all of this, that's enough work for now. Tuck this bonus thought away: There is a foodie world out there, and you have the key to open the door to embrace that foodie world the moment you're ready.

ready for more

If you've been incorporating the tools in the beginning of this book or in the previous paragraphs, you may be ready for more. Your next challenge is to believe that *food is not the enemy.* Food is simply food; it's neither inherently evil nor essentially virtuous. Your feelings about food and food allergies are the true challenge (or potential enemy). Once you're ready to change your feelings about food, then eating, dining at home, dining out, dating, social events, and traveling will all become much easier. Think of feeling at ease about food as your goal. Here are several ways to get closer to that goal.

Change the self-talk. Remember the voices we discussed in chapter 3 and in the section above. Those are the inner voices that say you're alone, you're scared, and food is evil. Those voices are normal, but the louder you allow them to become, the heavier your burden will feel. Quiet them, calm them, and replace them. Quiet them by recognizing when they're happening. The voices may be shouting at you because you're not listening. So listen. If you're in danger, heed the voices. If you perceive danger but none exists, move on to calming the loud voices. Tell yourself, "I'm okay." Repeat: "I'm okay." Or "I'm safe." Come up with your own calming sentence or a calming mantra. Borrow Master Shifu's mantra from the movie *Kung Fu Panda*: "Inner peace."

Once you're feeling calmer, your goal is to replace negative self-talk with positive statements. "Food is scary" becomes "Food is food. I may be feeling scared, but I know can take care of myself." The thought "I hate food" may become "I want to love food, and I'm going to find a way." The thought "I'm so different" can be transformed to "I have food allergies, and it's only one part of who I am." It takes time and practice; none of this happens overnight. Keep working on it.

Next, are you working your support system? If you haven't identified your safe friend yet, go do it or create one immediately. (Remember, a safe friend can be anyone: a close friend, a romantic partner, or a family member, or all three.) Don't delay, because with your safe friend by your side, you can expand your food-loving world. If you have a safe friend but don't seem to be reaping the full benefits, try to be more vulnerable in your conversations with him or her. Explain how you really feel (the most embarrassing parts you've been hiding—yes, those). You may be pleasantly surprised by the supportive reception from your identified safe friend. Also, with your safe person, you could come up with a dream list of things you'd like to do but have felt were off-limits because of your food allergies. Talk with your allergist about how to keep yourself safe; then, with your safe friend, go tackle some of those dreams together.

Next, you need some positive food images to replace the images of fear and loathing that you may have. Go to your local library, bookstore, or favorite online bookseller and find some books to help you transform your relationship to food. Self-help is not limited to books in that particular genre but exists in many forms. One of my food-allergy coaching clients loved *French Women for All Seasons* by Mireille Guiliano. She said it helped her to reconnect to the French way of extracting pleasure from food even after her diagnosis of food allergies and food intolerances. It's a brilliant idea. There are hundreds of wonderful food-related titles to help you connect.

The Spanish poet Pablo Neruda's *Selected Odes* about food are deceptively simple yet luscious. From "Ode to salt": "Dust of the sea, in you/the tongue receives a kiss/from ocean night." Read Neruda and get lifted; I feel lifted right now simply rereading it.

See some food movies, the kind that revel in food. Look at them as targets; you may be feeling rueful about your relationship to food right now, but becoming happier about that relationship is your target. Get some gluten-free ziti, spin some Louis Prima tunes, and make the timpano from *Big Night*. Cook a Chinese gluten-free banquet and watch *Eat Drink Man Woman*. Buy some allergen-safe chocolates and let them melt on your tongue as you watch *Chocolat*. Rent the German *Mostly Martha* or the American version *No Reservations* and get yourself a white apron and whisk as you create allergen-free masterpieces in your kitchen. Loudly slurp noodles as you watch the Japanese classic *Tampopo*. Do you love butter (or vegan buttery spreads)? *Julie & Julia* is simply bubbling over with buttery goodness. A lovable French rat who's a whiz in the kitchen is the cartoon star of *Ratatouille*. "Snap out of it!" and watch Cher's Oscar-winning performance in *Moonstruck*. (These make great date movies, too.) These are just some titles to get you started; your local library, Netflix, or iTunes will have more.

Watch some foodie television. There's everything from the pig-out *Man v. Food* to the encyclopedic Alton Brown's *Good Eats* on

some of my favorite allergen-friendly chocolate indulgences

Betty Crocker gluten-free mixes: www.bettycrocker.com/products/gluten-free-baking-mixes
Cherrybrook Kitchen mixes: http://cherrybrookkitchen.com
Divvies: Made to Share: www.divvies.com
Enjoy Life Foods: www.enjoylifefoods.com
Kinnikinnick: http://consumer.kinnikinnick.com

basic cable. I'm equal-opportunity when it comes to watching rebel Anthony Bourdain's globe-trotting and eating or "bizarre eats" Andrew Zimmern's globe-trotting and eating. The idea is to let yourself dream, be inspired, and reconnect to food as more than just fear.

Expand your diet. What are your food restrictions? List them. Now make another list of what you *can* eat. Now look at the "can eat" list and think about adding to it. How? Here's one example. Foods are classified into groups. Remember kingdom, phylum, class, order, family, genus, and species from Bio class? If you can eat from the broccoli family of vegetables, for example, there are several other cruciferous family vegetables that you can probably add (check first with your allergist or a registered dietitian well-versed in food allergies): cauliflower, horseradish, kale, collard greens, brussels sprouts, kohlrabi, broccoli romanesco, broccoli rabe, Chinese cabbage, napa cabbage, turnips, rutabaga, rocket (arugula), watercress, radishes, daikon, and even wasabi. You didn't know these are all related? They are. If you added one new cruciferous veggie per week, you'd have more than four months' worth of new food in your diet.

The world of food is huge, and there are lots of safe foods out there to try. With thousands of new allergy-friendly foods coming out, available not only in specialty markets but also in chain supermarkets, there is a larger supply of processed treats and goodies to try. I'm not advocating a diet filled with processed food, but trying out a new cookie once in a while as part of a balanced diet can't hurt. For example, if you desperately miss Oreos (that is, sandwich cookies) because you're wheat allergic or gluten intolerant, or were diagnosed with celiac disease, there are several reputable gluten-free manufacturers who make gluten-free sandwich cookies—enough for you to try one a week for the next several weeks and be in Oreo-like heaven.

eating well

Speaking of processed foods and eating your broccoli, part of deepening your relationship to food may include a new member of Team You: a registered dietitian. Part of the challenge of food allergies is eating well within a restricted diet. Eating well means enjoying a wide range of nutritionally balanced and flavorful foods in a variety of settings (home, school, work, and social events). Eating a varied diet plentiful in greens, legumes, grains, fats, and proteins applies to you even if you have to eliminate certain items from any of those food groups.

How to make those substitutions safely, how to read labels, and how to reduce possible contamination are all crucial and learnable skills. For many of my coaching clients who are just learning about their food allergies, I refer them to registered dietitians (RDs) who work specifically with food allergies or food intolerances. According to Marion Groetch, a senior dietitian at the Jaffe Food Allergy Institute of the Mount Sinai School of Medicine, "A dietitian is needed when eliminating milk or wheat; when eliminating more than one food; when having a tough time with avoidance; or when your primary care physician indicates there's evidence of nutritional inadequacies." RDs are a great resource for everyone—whose diet couldn't use a little tweaking?—but are especially critical for those of us with dietary restrictions.

Recently, I led a food-allergy coaching client through a food-reaction discovery process. An RD was a key element in the client's ultimate dietary success. Emma came to me looking for support to reach a proper diagnosis. She had seen an allergist for testing, a gastroenterologist for further testing, and an RD but had not gotten a definitive answer to why she was sick with stomachaches and an excessive number of bathroom trips a day. She had also received conflicting diagnoses as the root cause. Our first task together was to coordinate her Team Emma care. We role-played questions to ask each member of her team, and got the doctors to start talking with one another. Within a few weeks, Emma had a clearer direction from her team, and she noticed an obvious pattern in her food diary. Wheat products were giving her extreme stomachaches, and nothing was causing an allergic reaction. She brought this information to her RD, who assisted Emma further by helping her to eliminate wheat from her diet safely, expand her diet in a nutritionally sound way, and get back on track. Eating well involves more variables then just getting your fruits and veggies every day, especially if you have adverse reactions to food. A knowledgeable RD can help to ensure that your restricted diet expands in food-positive ways. (See chapter 9 for how to interview an RD and find one in your area.)

reconnect to food as a sensual experience

Once you're really working these strategies, add this to the mix: reconnecting to food as a sensual experience. As George Costanza on *Seinfeld* once said, "Food and sex, those are my two passions. It's only natural to combine them." Whether you're using food in the very literal sense of sensuality, like our friend George (who, as always, took it six steps too far), or simply allowing yourself to receive the sensory pleasure that food can provide, you may feel you're missing something if you aren't experiencing this aspect of nourishment. There are real concerns here, and they cannot be ignored. Perhaps you heard about the unfortunate English couple who decided to eat food off of each other during an intimate encounter, only to both have allergic reactions to the food and have to rush to the hospital. Precautions must be taken to ensure your safety, but then, by all means, dig in.

Expand your sensual and sensory skills to include the joyous aspects of eating: smell, looks, texture, and tastes (including the five flavors: sweet, salty, sour, bitter, and umami, or savory). You have a list of safe foods. If you don't, go back and make that list now, then work on it with a food-allergy coach, your allergist, or an RD. Then try this exercise. For example, if nondairy yogurt is your thing, treat yourself to the best of that thing and savor every bite. Savoring implies not scarfing it down in front of the TV or the computer or shoveling it out of the plastic tub with a plastic spoon. Try a nice bowl with actual flatware or even silverware. Add toppings, like fresh picked berries or golden flowing honey. (Yes, you can add allergen-friendly chocolate, too). What about trying a nondairy yogurt taste test? There are many delicious vegan, dairy-free, or low-lactose yogurt options, made with soy milk, rice milk, coconut milk, nut milk, or goat's milk. Buy a container of every brand you can find, taste each solo or with a friend, and discover your favorite one. You could even get a yogurt starter and make your own; play with flavors (I'm partial to coffee or caramel), textures (I like thick versus runny), and toppings (homemade nut-free granola is calling out to me). How about making nondairy frozen yogurt? The options are endless. Enjoying food sensuously is one of life's greatest pleasures; don't miss out.

how to love food without *loving* food

There's a line between having a healthy attachment to food and an unhealthy attachment to food. Many people in the food-allergic community who are in denial about food allergies believe that they have no attachment to food or the adverse effects it can have on their bodies; others, however, go in the opposite direction, way overboard, allowing food allergies to dominate all conversations, social activities, and brain space.

Some of you may have a specific negative history with food: compulsive eating, emotional eating, overeating, undereating, or bingeing and purging. Talking about creating a love of food may bring up old hurts or old behavioral patterns. If you fit into this category, you may think that a love of food is the last thing you need. For example, an Allergicgirl.com blog reader bravely e-mailed me with this concern:

> I developed an adult-onset shellfish allergy when I was about 25 (for which I carry an Epi-pen). I've been intolerant to eggs since childhood, too. About 10 days ago, I was given the results of my food allergy testing: I'm reactive to a ton of foods. Suddenly, I've been thrust into a totally new way of eating. Add to that, I've got a history of anorexia with a relapse only three years ago. These new restrictions are playing with my mind right now. I've worked so hard in recovery the last three years to make any food allowable, so now, being told that I must restrict, even if it's for a different/good reason, is hard to deal with. It's hard to wrap my head around it. I feel like I belong to a special category of crazy right now.

This reader has made the first great step: recognizing that food allergies may reactivate her anorexia. As she moves through the process of diagnosis toward acceptance, more feelings may arise. Anyone with a history of food abuse in any form must check in with not only a medical professional but also a qualified mental health professional who specializes in eating disorders. Add those professionals to your Team You, or revitalize previous professional relationships for short-term work. Even though you may feel like a "special category of crazy," you are not alone. There are many others with food allergies with histories like yours. Find them and connect with them.

support for those with a history of food-related disorders

Find support groups in your area through local hospitals, schools, or religious groups, or contact the following:

- American Psychiatric Association: www.psych.org
- American Psychological Association: www.apa.org
- National Association of Social Workers: www.socialworkers .org
- National Eating Disorders Association: www .nationaleatingdisorders.org
- National Institute of Mental Health: www.nimh.nih.gov/ index.shtml

the best is yet to come

If you've had food allergies a long time, you might think that you don't need this chapter at all. My questions to you are the following: Are you getting everything you want from your relationship to food? Are you going to work functions and having a great time and a great dinner, or are you avoiding the functions, begging off at the last minute? Are you going to social and family events but not eating or are afraid to eat and thus remain hungry and feeling unhappy and left out? How will an attitude shift, like believing that you're a foodie possibly help you?

I spent many years believing that no one could serve me something safe: no chef, no friend, no cousin—no one. At the time, I was right. I was feeling so marginalized, so restricted, that no one could have possibly helped me. Finally, tired of not trusting, believing that there must be something better, I challenged myself to take a mental leap to believing that this restaurant, that hostess, this caterer, or that friend would be able to feed me safely and well. That internal shift means that now, nine times out of ten, I do eat safely and well, everywhere: dining at home, dining out, going to work events or social functions, and traveling. I enact specific strategies to ensure safety, and I manage risk. But it all began with this mental shift: *I want more.*

If you had asked me five years ago whether I thought this was possible, I would probably have said, "It's all right, I'm fine. I don't need more." But I wasn't having as much fun. Yes, I was fine five years ago, but I'm better now. And I want you to be, too. If you're like me, and you've had food allergies a long time and you're fine where you are now, great. But perhaps it's time for a rediscovery. Think of Anne of *Anne of Green Gables* and her life affirming exuberance when she said, "Isn't it splendid to think of all the things there are to find out about? It just makes me feel glad to be alive—it's such an interesting world. It wouldn't be half so interesting if we know all about everything, would it? There'd be no scope for imagination then, would there?" If you want more, it's time for you to get it. What is your relationship to food right now, and how can you explore your relationship to food in a deeper, different way? How can you make your relationship to food more robust, more fulfilling, more interesting with a wider scope and, above all, more fun? I challenge you to go back through the middle section of this chapter and be honest with yourself about where you are and then dream about where you'd like to be.

create a love of food

Whether you're newly diagnosed or you've been coping with food allergies for what seems like forever, ask yourself: What do you want your relationship with food to be? I want mine to be easy, safe, unworrisome, unanxious, enjoyable, and not the focus of my life. Come up with some adjectives; go crazy, don't edit. Dream big, dream small—just dream. You don't have to be a foodie, or a food lover; you don't have to subscribe to food magazines, read food blogs, watch food shows, or learn a new foodie language. Just come up with something and expand your scope of food.

Being educated about food, about your diagnosis, about what can cause an allergic or adverse reaction in your body—and knowing where those foods are found, in which cuisines or which dishes—will greatly reduce your anxiety around food and help you to connect to food in a positive way. The point is to reduce any potential food-allergen fear by having the information you need to make informed choices about the appropriate level of safety in any situation and to create a positive new connection to food and nourishing your body in a healthy, satisfying way.

allergic girl's tasty tidbits

- A food-allergy diagnosis will forever change your relationship to food; however, you control that relationship.
- Recognize that because of food allergies, you have a passionate relationship to food. Embrace that passion as positive.
- If you're in the beginning of accepting food allergies, work your support system and your Team You.
- If you're ready for more, start to cultivate a love of food. Add new foods to your diet, tap into food culture, get back into the sensory experience of food.
- There's a distinct difference between loving food and *loving* food. Be sure you know the difference. If you have a history of eating disorders, check with a qualified mental health professional to help you through the transition.
- Just because you've had food allergies a long time doesn't mean there's nothing left to learn. Go deeper into that conversation with yourself.
- Ultimately, having a self-loving, positive relationship with food and your food allergies will help you to navigate the world with ease.

part three

in and of
the world

8

to be in the world and of the world

I have learnt how to live . . . how to be in the world and of the world, and not just to stand aside and watch.

—Sabrina Fairchild, *Sabrina*

One of my favorite Billy Wilder movies is *Sabrina*. It stars the elegant Audrey Hepburn playing Sabrina Fairchild, a chauffeur's daughter. Sabrina longingly observes the überrich Larrabees living their lavish life in a Long Island mansion. (Think F. Scott Fitzgerald's East Egg, but thirty years later.) In addition, she's hopelessly in love with David Larrabee, the playboy son, portrayed with rakish charm by William Holden. Humphrey Bogart plays the older, highly successful but less romantically desirable son, Linus.

143

As Sabrina comes of age, she's sent to cooking school in Paris as a diversion from David. While in Paris, she learns about cracking eggs with one hand—"Eet's all een zee wreest"—and about cooking a soufflé: "A woman happily in love, she burns the soufflé. A woman unhappily in love, she forgets to turn on the oven." Most significant, she learns "how to be in the world and of the world, and not just to stand aside and watch." Sabrina returns home a changed woman, receiving amorous attention from not one but both Larabee brothers.

To be in the world and of the world; to be inside your life, not watching it pass by or standing on the sidelines merely wishing you could join in; to participate in all that life has to offer; to be a contributor to your world and to the world—how *délicieux* is that? Sabrina's *cri de coeur* became my own as a food-allergic adult: how to stay safe and be both in and of the world. It's an excellent framework as we move through the last part of this book, putting everything together to become contributing food-allergic citizens in and of the world.

This chapter is your primer for being in and of the world. We will build on the core principles outlined in the first two parts of the book: the acceptance of your food-allergy diagnosis; the employment of a medical Team You; the identification or creation of emotional support from friends, family, and loved ones; and a positive connection to food. Having these core principles in place will give you the confidence you need to interact with those around you in a stronger, more positive way. If you don't have some of these structures in place yet, go back, reread the relevant sections, and start to enact them. (Do you need more support? Consider hiring a food-allergy coach to help you get on track.)

The primer concepts presented in this chapter are the underlying nuances, tones, and shades of thoughts, feelings, and actions that will help you to move through the nonallergic world with increased confidence. In the successive chapters, when we explore the hows, keep these primer concepts in the forefront of your mind.

rapport

Rapport is finding common ground with someone and making a connection. When you're the one with the special request, it's your job to make even a tiny link with the person who can help you to meet that need. Your two best tools are a genuine smile and an icebreaker, and you always have those on hand. First, smile; a real, genuine smile. Once that smile is returned you have a natural opportunity or opening. Extend a friendly gesture: a compliment ("That's a great tie/pin/watch/necklace."), a comment about the weather ("Whew, so glad the snow's over."), or something interesting in the local news (a happy or funny story, please) that sticks to the universals: babies, puppies, cupcakes, sunshine.

Many of us, when we're out of our safe zones, can feel extra anxious or worried about getting our food allergy needs met. That anxiety is often expressed as defensive anger or aggression, that is, not a smiley, happy face. For example, when I've been sharp, cutting, or brusque with restaurant servers or managers, it didn't help them to understand my needs more clearly; mainly, they just stayed out of my way. You want to attract assistance, not repel it. *Rapport* is from the French, meaning to "bring back." Think about that as you start to practice creating rapport: bring these people back to you, to what you need.

Take a moment in every situation to make a real and personal bond. Is someone at a deli making your sandwich with contaminated gloves? Make eye contact and flash a genuine smile, even when you're nervous, rushed, or annoyed. When you ask the sandwich handler to kindly change his or her gloves because you have food allergies, you'll be hard to resist. This doesn't have to be a big love affair, just a little niceness, some charm.

good enough trust

Creating rapport can eventually lead to feelings of trust. Although true, deep, and lasting trust is formed over time and through life's trials, all you need right now is a temporary trust—a good enough trust. A good enough trust is the next step, after a social connection the kind that typifies rapport, that you need to get your food allergic needs met out in the world.

Train yourself to see kind eyes and nonjudgmental warm hearts everywhere. Look for relaxed body language, good eye contact, and other signs that a person is listening and comprehending what you're saying, taking into account the seriousness of your food-allergy request. You can create good enough trust everywhere by recognizing the signs of a trustworthy individual. I find people every day with whom I create good enough trust, because I'm looking for them. It's that simple; perception becomes reality.

For example, during a business meeting with the chef of a Worry-Free Dinners partner restaurant, we were talking about food allergies, patrons, and trust. The chef said she was impressed that I was such an adventurous eater, given my allergy restrictions. I don't see myself as an adventurous eater, nor can I recall any other chef ever saying this to me. She thinks I'm adventurous because I trust her. I know that her restaurant is transparent about its ingredients and its methods of preparation. I know that she trains the servers personally, and everyone embraces the food-allergic patron. Because of that, I can say to her, "Sure, let's try that new dish, sounds great!" This is what establishing a good enough trust with a chef, for example, can do.

trust but verify

"Trust but verify" is a Russian axiom that former U.S. president Ronald Reagan was fond of employing. I've adopted it. Trust, when it comes to food allergies, doesn't mean "Oh, whew, now my life is in this complete stranger's hands, and I can take a brain nap" or "I'm so comfortable I can forgo the Steps" (as outlined below). It means that you trust others enough to do their job; *you* relay your needs to whoever should hear them, and *you* verify those needs every step of the way.

For instance, with the executive chef above, I trust her, but I don't say, "Sure, make me something" and then eat whatever she serves me. When she suggests trying something new, I remind her what my allergies are, and we go over the ingredients together. When the server brings the dish, I confirm with him or her that the dish is free of those allergens. I trust this chef, and I verify my needs. So create a good enough trust, and remember, it is your job to keep yourself safe.

food-allergy allies

One of the scarier scenarios I envision is the prospect of having a severe allergic reaction and being alone. In my mind it plays out like this: "I don't know anyone at this event or in this city, I did all of the Steps to ensure my safety, but there was a blunder, and now I'm feeling itchy and hivey and wheezy, and I know no one here." Of course, that panicky feeling only adds to an allergic reaction, or the fear of one, which definitely decreases the possibility of having a good time, be it a wedding, a holiday celebration, or an off-site work meeting.

In order to combat this, I enlist temporary food-allergy allies. We talked about creating allies within your family; this is a similar construct. The goal is to have someone, just one person, who knows that you have medical needs when you're in a foreign situation and that you may need assistance getting proper medical attention. That's it. Whether it's letting a hotel concierge know that I have some special needs or making friends with a restaurant manager, having someone who gets it makes dining or traveling (especially if solo) easier and safer.

Allies are everywhere; being open and honest about your needs uncovers them quickly. Seven times out of ten, when I tell servers at restaurants that I have severe food allergies, they tell me that their mothers, their lovers, or their best friends have food allergies, too. This happened just recently while I was dining alone at a new restaurant, sitting at the bar. When I told the bartender my food allergies, he said that his best friend also has severe nut allergies. He dines out with her all of the time, so he knew how scary it can be. "I will make sure you are taken care of," he said. That created enough of a connection, enough of an alliance, that if something were to happen while sitting at his bar, I would be able to say to this bartender, "I need some assistance," and he would be motivated to help. An ally is someone with whom you've created some rapport and with whom there's an element of trust, just a glimmer—that's all you need. This is really for a just-in-case scenario. Most likely you'll enjoy your meal and move on with your life. But "just in case" can happen at any time, and allies are a plus to have in your proverbial back pocket.

ally, not savior

Having said that, keep this in mind: Food-allergy allies aren't ever responsible for your safety. You are, always. Remember Vivi, the food-allergy deputy (see chapter 5). You can deputize food-allergy allies on the go, but you are always the sheriff. Someone on-site who knows about your needs while you're dining or traveling will decrease your anxiety and increase the chance that if something happens, you will have support in place to get you what you need if you can't get it yourself, like a hospital trip or an emergency call.

For example, the first destination wedding I went to after college was in a small town outside Los Angeles. I went for the weekend, flying by myself and staying in a hotel solo, and I knew only the bride and the groom. My ally became the manager of the hotel restaurant, where I ate by myself for two nights. He made sure to take care of me; he checked on me several times while I dined, sent over a glass of wine, and generally made himself available. My meals were delicious, I had no issues, and it was good to know that someone had my back.

What happens if you don't create an ally? Nothing. You can take care of yourself; if there's an emergency, you're prepared. It's simply some insurance.

do the steps

It seems like an obvious directive: do the Steps. But I have a hunch that a fair number of you are thinking, "I already do some steps. I already call ahead. I already talk to the managers or the caterers, and all I get is the eye roll, or they pity me. Or I end up screaming at them until they get it right. That's just how it is." There is definitely a high percentage of eye rollers and pitiers out there, and there always will be. But I see that only 10 percent of the time; 90 percent of the time it's all fine, dandy, friendly, and safe. What's the trick? There are no tricks, just incorporation of these primer concepts into some clearly defined actions and behaviors, that is, doing the Steps.

There are plenty of food-allergy blogs and Web sites that will tell you to do X, Y, and Z when going to a restaurant, for example: call ahead, talk with manager, talk with server, double check, and so forth. The difference here is not merely doing the X, Y, and Z but putting everything we've explored so far into *how* you talk with the restaurant manager, for example. The acceptance of your diagnosis and how that makes you feel about yourself; knowing how to take care of yourself in an emergency and the confidence that affords; the support of loved ones; and a readiness to expand your allergic world; putting all of those thoughts, feelings, and support in combination with the actions I'm going to outline in the next sections will bring you positive results in getting your needs met where ever, whenever.

If you've had food allergies a long time, and you feel like you already do your own food allergy procedures, but with mixed results, try tackling your usual steps with what Zen Buddhists call a beginner's mind. Approach my suggestions with an attitude of openness and enthusiasm, without preconceived outcomes, as a beginner would. For those of us who have had food allergies for a lifetime, we've had so many years of negative experiences that trying to be like a food-allergy virgin sounds impossible. This isn't about erasing the past; it's about knowing that you have options. Consider giving yourself a fresh start by releasing the need for a prescribed result; make your goal learning and positivity, and see what happens.

Be Prepared

I coach clients and Worry-Free Dinner members every day about what it means for a food-allergic person to be prepared. There are the basics: having lifesaving medications on your person at all times, knowing how and when to use them, listening to your body for signs of distress, gathering support around you, engaging with the world in a positive way, and setting your mental stage to allow yourself to engage and have fun.

There are additions to those basics: having backup plans, having safe snacks (in your purse, backpack, suitcase, or briefcase), or even eating a little something before you go out. The more prepared you are mentally, physically, and medically, the more options that are open to you. Everyone loves options, and when your diet is restricted, you can feel optionless. Being prepared will help to open up options you may not have seen before.

Of course, the worst usually happens when we are least prepared. I interviewed the Intelliject epinephrine autoinjector inventors Eric and Evan Edwards about their close call, which is part of why they invented the device. Here's the account from their Web site:

> Evan's most recent anaphylactic reaction from an accidental ingestion of nuts mixed with hummus happened while at a northern Virginia restaurant. Within minutes, his lips and throat began to swell and his body mounted a systemic allergic reaction. He didn't have an epinephrine auto-injector with him. Thankfully, Evan was immediately rushed to a local hospital by ambulance, receiving epinephrine to combat the anaphylactic reaction just in time.

Where was Evan's emergency epinephrine autoinjector? In my interview with the brothers for Healthcentral.com, Evan clarified, "I had left my epinephrine injector in my car at home; we had taken our friends' car to the restaurant and I had forgotten to grab it." Evan was lucky, we've all read stories about people who didn't have a hospital nearby and weren't so lucky.

Manage Your Expectations

Not every situation can be, or should be, tailored to your food-allergic needs. You'll often just have to make the best of a situation while staying safe. Is your office taking everyone on a hayride and apple-picking trip as a bonding activity? If you have hay fever and oral allergy syndrome to apples during fall, this might be a complete disaster for you, and corporate headquarters probably isn't going to change the whole event to suit your needs. Are you attending a second cousin's bridal shower at which you will know no one? Is it possible to get in touch with the best friend who's throwing the event and talk with her about your food allergies? Yes. Is it less stressful to eat before you go? Probably. If you have to attend a work event at a Japanese restaurant and you're fish-allergic, should you demand that they serve you a nonfish meal? You could, but they probably won't have many safe options for you, and you'll end up stuck and starved.

It is not necessary for you to be able to dine safely in every situation; sometimes it's easier to bring your own food or eat beforehand. Safety and fun are the goals, so look at the options and make the smart decision for right now. Manage your expectations about what can and should be done to accommodate your needs in individual situations.

Envision the Outcome

Mahatma Gandhi said, "Just put forth a clear enough request, and everything your heart desires must come to you." Isaac Newton said something similar in his third law of motion: Every action has an equal and opposite reaction. The character Guinan on *Star Trek: The Next Generation* said, "When a man is convinced he's going to die tomorrow, he'll probably find a way to make it happen." Every few years there's a new book craze around some version of the law of attraction. However you want to view it, it's a truism: you get out what you put in. I have coached hundreds of clients on this point alone.

When you approach an event thinking, "They're going to take great care of my needs" instead of "This is never going to work," there's a marked difference in outcome. Part of the difference is your facial expression—you know, the one that gets you nowhere fast, the this-is-going-to-be-a-disaster face: squinty eyes, stern eyebrows, turned-down mouth, and tight lips, accompanied by the body language of anxious energy, a rigid stance, and clenched fists. Now try going anywhere with an I-know-they're-going-to-make-me-something-yummy-and-safe face, smiling broadly, while you have a relaxed body posture and seem confident and flexible. It makes a real difference when you try an expression of confidence and joy. Envision that your food-allergic needs will be met, and let that register on your face. Watch what happens.

Realize That No One's Listening

Most people are more concerned with "Does my dress look all right?" or "Is my hair doing something funny?" or "I have a huge pimple on my nose" than with listening to someone else give a food-allergy list and order to a server. "People aren't really watching or listening to what you're doing—eating or not eating, ordering or not ordering. People are usually most concerned with what they are doing, eating, or not eating. With that in mind, go about your business.

Here's an example: On a blind double date for dinner, I arrived early and spoke with the restaurant manager. He reassured me that he understood the seriousness of the situation and would make sure that "certain foods didn't touch my dishes." He also said he would have the chef go through the menu and indicate which items were safe for me. As we were being seated, the manager found me and said that the waitress had been briefed and would go over my menu choices at the table.

Very quietly, while the people at my table were laughing and drinking, the waitress came over to my chair and went through the menu that the chef had designed for me. We reviewed the ingredients, preparations, and substitutions. I gave her my order, and she said she'd be back in a moment for everyone else's. My blind date turned to me and said, "So what are the specials?"

See? No one was listening.

Use Frame Shifting, Focus, and Humor

Three tools to have in your primer concept shed at all times are frame shifts, maintaining your focus, and a sense of humor.

Frame shifting. This is partly the glass-half-full axiom and partly singer Johnny Mercer's "accentuate the positive" dictum. It's about shifting perspective, challenging yourself to see any positive within any negative. For example, do you feel awkward bringing your safe food to a catered event? There was a piece in the February 19, 2010, *New York Times* about folksinger Judy Collins. She brings her food with her everywhere. She's not allergic, but she has a strict diet. As a working artist, she said, she "only eat[s] what I'm supposed to be eating, because in this line of work, you have to live like an athlete." Use that as a frame shift: you are a *food-allergy athlete*, and you can eat only what you're supposed to be eating. Hazzah, frame shift!

Focus. A national or religious holiday, a family celebration, and a work event are not about you personally. So, *focus on the focus of the event.* You are not the focus during a religious event or holiday, nor should your food allergies be the focus of the office quarterly sales meeting. Keep the focus on why you are there. A friend's birthday? A bridal shower? A work colleague's going-away party? Do your best to get your needs met simply and easily, or make the determination to preempt (by eating beforehand or elsewhere or by bringing food) and go and enjoy.

Humor. There's humor in everything, from the sublime to the truly ridiculous. A restaurant that sends me a supposedly different order of pancakes when all the cook did was simply scrape the nuts off the original batch, thinking I wouldn't notice—that's not merely poor service, a lack of awareness about allergies, and dangerous, it's outrageous. I have to laugh and not touch what they've served me, of course.

Having a sense of humor isn't about not taking your food-allergy needs seriously; it's about seeing the lightness while you're ensuring your safety. Find something funny; it will lighten your psychological and physical load. The more accepting you become of your diagnosis and the more confident you feel about being able to take care of yourself, the more you will see the inherent silliness (even absurdity) in many food-allergy-related situations.

If you don't have a sense of humor about your dietary restrictions, think about the reasons. Are you feeling angry, marginalized, hurt, confused, or unable to take care of your needs? If you're not there yet, tuck this away for when you're ready. Humor is an excellent tool to have in your food-allergy coping-mechanisms toolbox. Bonus: If you can laugh when you get the eye roll or the pity look, the power of those expressions evaporates.

contradictions: yes and no

It may seem as though everything I just wrote is contradictory: have trust, but not too much; have an ally, but don't rely on him or her; take steps, but know the limitations; engage with those around you, but realize that no one's listening; envision your outcome, but have a beginner's mind; assume that everyone should be able to service your needs, but don't think that every event can be tailored to you; and take your needs seriously, but laugh and the world laughs with you.

Perhaps they are contradictory, but they do dovetail. As you become more adept at moving through this process, you'll find the place between too much and not enough. With practice, you'll learn how to internalize the nuances—when to be more forceful and when to laugh, when to trust, and when to walk away. Try the techniques in the following chapters; I use them and teach them to my private coaching clients and during Worry-Free Dinners events, and I've found them to be highly effective. With these primer concepts, get ready to go out into the world and make it yours.

allergic girl's primer concepts

- Acceptance of your diagnosis, a great Team You and support system, and a positive connection to food will increase your overall confidence.
- You have basic interpersonal tools at your disposal at all times and for various situations and scenarios.
- Create rapport and good enough trust; however, always verify your needs.
- Food-allergy allies are everywhere, but remember that you are your best first responder in an emergency.
- Take the precautions outlined in this book and always be prepared.
- Manage expectations, but also envision positive outcomes.
- If you feel self-conscious about asking for what you need, remember: most people aren't paying attention.
- Frame shift, maintain focus, and find the funny: these are lifelines.
- Ultimately, find a balance among all of these invaluable tools, depending on the situation and where you are now.

9

the home-court advantage

What are you doing?"

"What do you mean? I'm getting a place setting for my takeout."

"But didn't they give you paper plates and plastic forks?"

"Yes, but it's nicer to eat on real plates, right?"

"Of course, and you know you're welcome to anything in my home. But didn't you just say that you got miso-encrusted salmon?"

"Yeah . . . and . . ."

I had to laugh. My safe friend Casey was over for dinner. We dine together weekly, she knows all about my allergies, and she's usually very considerate. But now, here, in my kitchen, she was getting some of *my* plates and *my* silverware for her take-out *salmon* dinner. I never put limits on what anyone eats, whether near me at the same table, before we get together, or even in my home. Food is to be enjoyed, and, as we've discussed, food is just food. But I didn't necessarily want Casey dishing up miso-marinated salmon from the local high-end Japanese restaurant on my plates, either, especially since I don't own a dishwasher and salmon is particularly oily. So I just looked at Casey and smiled. And waited.

"Oh, my gosh. The salmon! Of course—I'll use the plates and forks they gave me. I didn't even think. So sorry."

We had a good giggle, and then we had dinner, Casey with her salmon on a paper plate, me with my homemade vegan lentil soup in a ceramic bowl.

home sweet home

Would it surprise you to know that I often allow my Kryptonites, nuts and fish, into my home? When ex-boyfriend Henry ordered the eel and salmon-skin sushi, it was cool. Chinese cashew chicken take-out for Danielle, no problem. New friend Kate brought walnut lace cookies as a house gift. No panic here: walnut lace cookies and Earl Grey tea coming right up.

Do you think I'm playing with allergen fire or consorting with the food-allergen enemy by allowing my allergens into my home? I'm enacting a decision I made about how I will interact with food in a safe and positive way. That decision is this: I am in the world and of the world, the whole world—including tree nuts and fish. The world is filled with things that may cause me harm. Protecting myself from food-allergen harm is my job; it's your job, too. I let my allergens into my orbit because I have to; they are everywhere in the outside world, regardless of my feelings about them. It's best to make an informed decision about how to handle being around them in the world, and that starts in my home.

Do you feel nervous about having your allergens in your home? This is a perfect time for a visit to your allergist or medical Team You. (See the sample questions later in this chapter.) Discuss the real risks, your cross-contamination fears, how to keep your kitchen safe, and your emergency plans.

questions to consider

How would you handle the prior scenario? If you were allergic to salmon, would you allow it in your home? How would you handle a conversation about banned foods or allowed foods with room-mates, family members, or romantic partners? How do you feel about your allergens just being around you? Where is your current anxiety level? Where would you like it to be?

We're going to examine several typical scenarios and circum-stances, focusing on making informed choices about the appro-priate level of safety in your home. The goal here is to have a life while staying safe. Although the scenarios will change and there will be challenges in each, the basic focus will remain the same. Go with where you are now. If that's a completely allergen-free home, that's okay, do it. If it's having college roommates who understand, great, help them to understand your needs. Maybe it's a husband who cooks allergen-free food for you and consumes your allergens only when he's out with his buddies—super, talk with him about your feelings and how you can stay safe. Let's look at some typical scenes in these types of situations and see what your options are.

Home Is Where the Stomach Is

Alex Désert of the ska band Hepcat sang, "Where your heart is, is where you'll find your home." I would add that home is the dwelling where you spending large amounts of time when you're not at work; where you have all of your stuff; and where you do a significant amount of dining and snacking and are in and around a kitchen. Maybe you're in college, in your dorm room or in off-campus housing. Maybe you've left college and, like many new graduates, have moved back home with your family. Maybe you're not at home but living with roommates after college. Perhaps you're living alone or with an intimate partner. The concept of home includes being cozy, warm, and safe. So you need to figure out what that means for you, wherever you are now.

Team You and Dining at Home

Whether you're heading off to college or moving overseas for a new job, checking in with your allergist will help you to get there safely. Talk to the allergist about what he or she recommends for your personal safety at home: symptoms to watch out for in case you have an allergic reaction, prescriptions for emergency medications, and an emergency plan and sharing it with housemates or loved ones. If you've been putting off a visit to the allergist, go now. The following are sample questions to ask an allergist about staying safe while at home:

- Can you please clarify my allergy diagnosis as it pertains to eating at home?
- What are your best suggestions for staying safe, given the severity of my reactions?
- Should I remove all allergens entirely?
- Would I be safe enough if I allowed allergens in my home and made sure that they were stored separately and that cross-contamination was avoided?
- When I shop for food, what should I watch out for on labels?
- What do you think about "May contain" labels? Can I still consume those foods with a minimum of risk?
- What do you think about airborne allergens? Am I at risk? What can I do to protect myself?

- What are the real dangers? What's reasonable?
- Can we go over my emergency plan—what to do when and what medications to take and how?

The more honest your questions, the better you will be able to deduce real risk versus irrational fears. Are you still feeling shy about talking with a doctor? Reread chapter 2 and then practice with your safe person before going; talk through what you need to ask. It gets easier with practice, so practice and then go to the doctor. You need this information—make certain you get it.

Nutrition Counseling

As we explored in chapter 8, a registered dietitian (RD) is an excellent addition to your Team You to ensure that you are getting adequate nutrition when you're dining at home. Ideally, your medical Team You members should confer with one another so that everyone is on the same page. Ask your allergist or your general practitioner for an RD recommendation; that way he or she will be someone your doctor already knows and trusts.

When you see your RD, be clear and up front about your pre-existing dietary restrictions and what kinds of assistance you need. You're looking for an RD who's very knowledgeable about food allergies and food substitutions. Do not employ any medical professional or health professional who is not an expert in the area you need most. Remember, Team You works for you. As suggested by Marlisa Brown, author of *Gluten-Free, Hassle Free*, when you're looking for an RD who is knowledgeable in food allergies, ask the following questions of the RD or the staff before making an appointment:

- What percentage of your patients have been medically diagnosed with food allergies?
- What are the typical food allergens and food-allergy patients that you have worked with?

- Will you be able to develop a meal plan that takes into account my likes and dislikes as well as my food allergies?
- Will you be able to provide me with a list of appropriate substitutions for my food allergies?

Marion Groetch, a senior dietitian at the Jaffe Food Allergy Institute of the Mount Sinai School of Medicine, suggests the following questions for RDs:

- Have they received any specific training in food allergies (attended ADA- or AAAAI-sponsored or approved conferences or completed any continuing education courses)?
- How do they update their food-allergy knowledge?

These are all excellent questions that will help you to determine, before you make an appointment, if a particular RD is the right person for you. Seeing an RD for a consultation is especially helpful for those who are new to food allergies. Are you heading off to college? That's a perfect time to check in and talk about how to eat when you're away from home. Are you making a voluntary dietary shift, such as becoming a vegan or a vegetarian? Check with a knowledgeable RD to make sure you are getting the nutrition you need. (Contact the American Dietetic Association, www.mypyramid.gov or www.eatright.org, 800-877-1600, to find qualified RDs in your area.)

dining at college

Your college years are a time of immense learning, on all levels. They're also an opportune time to try out new strategies, new selves, and new ways of being and interacting. For those with a medical condition like food allergies, this is a time when what's been working at home is put to the test and challenged and new pathways are formed.

Are you already overwhelmed? Reframe and channel those but-
terflies into your first adult challenge. Practice how to work within
a typically bureaucratic system to get your needs met. The prize
is the satisfaction of learning how to get what you need without
your family's intervention. It's all fantastic rehearsal for when you
enter the world stage. Here are some questions to consider discussing with your family, your family doctor and your allergist, your
friends, and even yourself:

- What is your ideal living situation?
- What's your ideal dining location?
- Are you a budding chef who wants to cook in the dorm, or
  do you favor take-out and microwaved meals?
- Would dining hall food with allergy modifications by
  an allergy-knowledgeable kitchen staff be acceptable, or is
  your allergy severe enough to warrant separate food cooked
  in a separate facility?

Your answers will inform how you move forward.

The Dining Hall

After you've chosen your dream institution, search for "Dining"
on the college Web site (very often under "Student Life"). Several
colleges and universities, large and small, public and private, have
food-allergen policies already in place; some have gone as far as
to create allergen-free or peanut-free dining halls. Reach out to
the head of dining, the facilities manager, or the supervisor (the
information should also be on the college Web site) and have a
conversation about how the system works. Be friendly, polite, and
upbeat. Make this person your new best friend.

Here's a sample discussion (by e-mail or phone):

> Hi! I'm Sloane Miller, and I'm in the incoming class
> of 2015. I have severe food allergies to tree nuts and
> salmon. I'm looking for some more information about

dining on campus. I see you have a program in place; could you tell me more about it? If I have more questions, whom do I ask? Is there one person on-site in the dining hall whom I should talk to? What if I have an extra-special request—is that something you can handle? Thank you so much.

When you arrive on campus, walk over to this person's office or ask to meet him or her in the kitchen for a tour. Introduce yourself by name to the kitchen staff. Make friends. Smile. Be gracious. Yes, really, you can do it. Are you feeling shy? If your parents helped to move you in, even though it's a hectic day, make it a priority to look for the head of dining together. Are you feeling shy but you don't want your parents there, holding your hand? After you've made a friend or two on campus, have those friends join you while you go and introduce yourself.

How does this help? I knew the name of every cafeteria worker who ever served me lunch, from grade school through graduate school. Because I had special needs and requests, I introduced myself, asked staff their names, and gave them mine. I never had an issue in the lunch line. (This was decades before the concept of peanut-free tables.) Cafeteria servers are people you see every day, so creating rapport should be easy: start with a smile and an introduction.

The benefit of this connection during college, for example, was a prized corner piece of lasagna or a saved portion of the vegan lentil bake from the night before. These cafeteria servers never minded when I asked to see the label on a package or asked about the ingredients of a dish. Once, when I was ill at college, the cafeteria server went into the kitchen and made me a special honey and lemon hot toddy. Why? Out of the thousands of students who passed through those halls, I was one of a select few who had made a connection with her. So make a connection; it will serve you well.

On-Site RDs

Many colleges now have RDs on staff to help with general nutrition as well as special dietary requirements. Use this resource; reach out to these RDs to discuss your needs and create a plan. Here's a sample first contact (by e-mail or phone) with a university or college staff RD, who will know the intricacies of that particular system:

> Hi! I'm Sloane Miller, and I'm in the incoming class of 2015. I have severe food allergies to tree nuts and salmon. I can send you a letter from my allergist if you'd like further information. I'm looking for more information about dining with food allergies while on campus. I see there are food-allergen programs already in place, but I'm hoping you could help me navigate the system. Where can I get the safest food? Whom should I talk to within dining services? Is there one point person? Is one dining hall easier to deal with than another? What protocols are in place in the kitchen? Any information you could offer would be great. Thank you!

Follow-up is essential. If the RD gives you names of dining hall people with whom to talk, make sure to contact them. When you get on campus, drop by the RD's office for a quick hello so he or she can put a face to your name. If you need additional help during your time on campus, this will be invaluable to you, for you now have an on-campus food-allergy ally.

The Dean Dialogue

If your chosen college or university doesn't have a food-allergen protocol in place yet, you'll need to get in there and create one. This will be the first of many conversations about your needs and the ability of another person or an institution to meet that need. The sooner you start having these conversations with confidence, the better. Connect to your food allergy needs without shame, embarrassment, and apology. Communicate those needs clearly, assertively, and graciously. Recognize that you have options. If you think that your dining hall or university won't be able to accommodate you, know this: there's always a way. It's usually a matter of finding either the right person with whom to talk or creating the solution yourself.

Don't delay this conversation or put it off until the morning before you leave for college. As soon as you accept a place in the incoming class, call and have a conversation about your needs and the staff's ability to meet those needs. Because food allergies have been on the rise, it is likely that you are not the first student who has requested some extra attention from dining services or a dispensation to cook in the dorm. Nevertheless, make that connection.

Go straight to the top. Contact the dean of students, the dean of your college, or the president's office by phone or e-mail—or show up in person. Create rapport, extend good enough trust so that these people will be able to help you, and envision a positive outcome. Engage in a friendly dialogue; you're looking for information here, not being demanding or aggressive about your needs. Be respectful, tactful, and precise. State who you are, what your immediate needs are, and how, ideally, you'd like them met. Be prepared to offer solutions, not merely state what isn't available. These are the same strategies I encourage you to employ throughout your life, so start now and get some good practice. Here's an example:

> Hello! My name is Sloane Miller, and I'm in the incoming class of 2015. I have severe food allergies to tree nuts and salmon. I can send you a letter from my allergist if you'd like. I'm looking for more information about

dining on campus. I didn't see any information about any food-allergy programs in place in your on-campus dining facility. However, perhaps I missed something. Do you have protocols in place? If yes, great! What are they? If not, how has dining services handled these types of requests in the past? My concern is mainly about cross-contamination in the campus kitchen, ingredients, recipes, and dishes. (Alternatively: My allergy is so severe I need to have access to a kitchen to make my own food. What options are available to me?) Let's find a solution together so I can stay safe while eating on campus.

A Local Team You

If you're leaving home to go away to college, you need a Team You in your new location. Talk with your family doctor or allergist; either one may have a colleague near your college or university. When you get to campus, check in with the campus health service. Find the local hospital and learn the route to get there fast. Find a local doctor to write prescriptions for emergency allergy medications. Get this out of the way the first week that you arrive, before classes start; do not wait for an emergency.

College Roommates or Housemates

In my sophomore, junior, and senior years, I lived in a house that had a full kitchen. Since I had a lot of housemates, and they all had frequently visiting friends, boyfriends, and girlfriends, I quickly surmised that sharing a fridge or using communal pots and pans was going to be a hotbed of fights, lies, and drunken excuses. So I eliminated risk by keeping a little fridge in my room. I also had a small cabinet in which I stored a pot, a pan, sponges and dishwashing liquid, mixing bowls, dishes, and flatware, enough for two people (or one person who felt lazy about doing her dishes). Everything was kept in my room, and everything was clean at all times—vermin are not the guests you want. I cooked daily. I made pies, soups, stews, tea breads, and jams. I made these while my housemates were out of the house and I had the kitchen to myself. If you want to hash it out with your housemates, see the next section for sample dialogue about how to help them understand the seriousness of your food-allergy needs, keeping in the back of your mind that it's your job, not theirs, to keep you safe. Assess the reality of your needs and your roommate situations and manage your risk.

College Boyfriends and Girlfriends

Another potential difficulty is the college boyfriend or girlfriend. Review chapter 6 and practice talking to your date about food allergens. By the time this person has become closer, like a steady, he or she will know about this part of you. In college, however, there are many variables outside your control. Again, it is vital to know the severity of your allergies, to have a local allergist on hand, to have your medications up-to-date and on your person, to let your new friend know how to use it, and to have made some initial decisions about your basic needs.

During college, I stretched my food abilities. I was already a full-fledged foodie by then, and an ovo-lacto vegetarian. This would all come in very handy my senior year of college abroad. My British boyfriend, Rudyard, was tall, sporty, brilliant, and funny. He also had a very adventurous palate: the smellier the cheese, the moldier the haggis (a Scottish dish made with animal organs), the slimier the organ meat, the better. He was very proud of the one dish he could cook: kaiserschmarrn, which is an Austrian sweet pancake, topped with fruits. It was delicious, but between the two of us, I was the cook and he was the guy who was led by his stomach. Our first date was at my house for Sloane-made banana bread, apricot preserves, and tea. Well into our relationship, I created an authentic Mexican lunch for him and his best friend. However, the high point of our culinary bond was when Rudyard told me that he simply loved liver with apples and onions, never believing that I'd cook it for him, since I was a vegetarian. I had no problems cooking everything; I just couldn't (or in this case, chose not to) eat everything. I did some recipe research at the library and surprised him later that week with his favorite meal. He was still crowing about it years later. For me, this was a way in, being in and of the world, engaging with the foods that he loved, even though I wouldn't consume them.

Cutting through Nut Fears

After my senior year abroad, I lived and worked in London for six months. I was a counter girl at an English chain of vegetarian restaurants in Covent Garden. The menu was a combination of vegan and vegetarian dishes, using only whole grains, vegetables, fruits, nuts, and seeds. One of my duties was to prepare the tea cakes, which were nut-based. Walnut bars, walnut bread, walnut loaf—I was surrounded. My understanding from my allergist was that I had to ingest the allergen to have a response. With that tucked away in the back of my mind, I wore double gloves and cut the cakes slowly and carefully so as to minimize nut debris. I made sure I cut in an open area, with lots of ventilation. My medications were nearby in the staff lockers.

And guess what? I had no issues, not even once. Although I would never recommend that you handle your allergens in this manner, my experience of working with nuts taught me an important lesson about my irrational fears versus the reality of my severe tree-nut allergies: I could be around nuts and not have a reaction.

A 2004 study in the *Journal of Allergy and Clinical Immunology* backed up my empirical data (what I learned was through trial and error, but I had no error):

> After [the subjects had engaged in] hand washing with
> liquid soap, bar soap, or commercial wipes, [the peanut

allergen] was undetectable. . . . The major [peanut aller-gen] is relatively easily cleaned from hands and tabletops with common cleaning agents and does not appear to be widely distributed in preschools and schools. We were not able to detect airborne allergen in many simulated environments.

This is just one study, and many more need to be done; how-ever, I hope this underscores how important it is to know what your needs are and precisely why you need to talk to your allergist about the severity of a possible reaction. Armed with the correct information, you can further ascertain what steps must be taken in your home for optimal quality of life and safety.

postcollege

After your college years, you will have plenty of new living situ-ations to deal with: moving back home, living with roommates, or living with a romantic partner or spouse. All of these situations will necessitate open and honest conversations about your needs, understanding and compassion, and education, for yourself and those around you on how to keep allergen-free.

Living at Home

Many college graduates move home for a year or so after college while they plan their next steps. Especially in a trying economy, it's not always practical to move out on your own. Sit down and have an adult conversation about your food allergies and your family's needs. This conversation will be necessary if your family members have been dining happily on your allergens while you were away. It will be less necessary if they have continued to keep the home allergen-free.

As a family, decide what works for everyone and what makes the most sense. Here are some questions to consider, adapted from the Food Allergy Initiative (www.faiusa.org):

- How severe is the allergy?
- If you were to completely eliminate problem foods, how difficult would it be for the other people in your house?
- How will your decision affect the overall quality of your home life?
- If you do decide that it's best to ban problem foods at home, how do you deal with the issue when you leave your home and go into the world?
- Is allergy-proofing your home doable or desirable?

Returning as an adult to your parents' home is a perfect time to exercise some of the new skills you've developed. Engage in a conversation with your family about what works for everyone now. Respect that the family may want to keep your allergens in the home. How will you stay safe? Work through your feelings and thoughts as well as what your allergist or medical Team You recommends.

Roommates or Housemates

My food-allergy coaching client Ben and I worked together to create a listing to find roommates who would understand his food allergies and respect them in the common areas of the house. As Ben felt more confident about his needs, he feel better about making those needs known up front, which eliminated confusion later. Ben's level of openness set the stage for continued excellent communication with his roommates. Here's part of his roommate listing:

> As a foodie, I love sharing meals with friends and roommates. One thing to note: I have a severe allergy to nuts, and the apartment I move into would have to be a

nut-free zone. My allergy means that even coming into physical contact with nuts could produce an allergic reaction that leads to death. Having a nut-free apartment eliminates the risk of consuming nuts, as well as the risk of a reaction from physical contact. I'm happy to clarify by e-mail or over the phone.

Through this brave advertisement, Ben found roommates who became food-allergy allies and even safe people.

When Mistakes Happen with Roommates

Ben told me the following story about roommates and label reading—a potential mistake that was effortlessly corrected.

My new roommates were totally jazzed about having me join them. They hadn't had much personal experience with food allergies but were eager to learn and very willing to make our apartment nut-free. A few days after moving in, I walked into the kitchen and was caught off guard by the unmistakable whiff of something not right. I was feeling unhinged but worked hard to keep my demeanor pleasant.

"What are you making?"

"Pasta."

"Oh? What kind of sauce?" I asked nonchalantly.

"Oh, you know, tomato, basil, olive oil . . ."

I smelled another ingredient that she wasn't naming. And I was impatient.

"Are there any nuts in this dish?"

"The only seasoning I put in is zaatar."

This Middle Eastern spice mixture is usually composed of sumac, thyme, sesame seeds, and nuts.

"Can I see that package of zaatar again?"

She handed it to me with a bit of uncertainty. We had both inspected the zaatar packaging the day before; two pairs of eyes had scanned the ingredients and thought that it was nut-free. In spite of our apparent care, there it was, third from the top, right behind salt: nuts. My roommate apologized and assured me that she'd take it to work first thing in the morning. [It was] Very kind of her to take responsibility, but in this case it was definitely a shared burden. We'd both failed to take note. The wonderful thing is that she proposed concrete action steps to mitigate any further risk. She immediately scoured the pans clean and put all the dishes away. Even though we'd delved into a risky situation, my new roomie was a certified safe person.

Ben had set up an open and nonjudgmental line of communication between himself and his housemates. At the outset, he explained his needs with confidence and remained patient while his housemates got up to speed.

Living with a Romantic Partner

Kyle Dine told me the following story about how he and his fiancée, who has celiac disease, negotiate their home space:

> I grew up with peanut butter in the house and am comfortable with my allergens being present. My fiancée and I trust each other to take the necessary precautions to prevent cross-contamination in our apartment. Regarding keeping a safe shared space, we are both very conscious of keeping a clean kitchen. I use a separate cutting board for when I'm cutting bread and am constantly cleaning the kitchen counter for crumbs. Whenever she prepares something for herself which contains something to which I'm allergic, I ask her to just do a thorough job of cleaning all of the prep space, utensils, and dishes.

Several years ago, my boyfriend at the time, Henry, often stayed over for several days in a row, cooking for the two of us. He was generally a healthy eater—lots of veggies and fish, tree nuts, and salads—and he would often order fish soup from the local Chinese restaurant for an afternoon snack on weekends. Without my asking, he would eat directly from the take-out containers and brush his teeth thoroughly afterward.

As I've already noted, my decision to be in the world and of the world meant that I allow allergens in my home in a safe way, and Henry used safe protocols. We had frank discussions about my dietary needs very early in our dating life, and even on our first date he knew I was food-allergic, so he suggested a well-known organic restaurant that was conscious of food allergies. Months into our relationship, he remained that mindful of my food-allergic needs in my home and took it upon himself to act with the utmost care around me. Overall, he was a safe person regarding my food allergies throughout our romantic relationship, and even now as friends he remains mindful.

Both of these examples of food-allergy supportive romantic partners are fairly straightforward: "I'm allergic to this, so let's take these precautions. Once that's done, we can smooch. Thanks!" With intimate partners and relationships, however, it may not always be this easy. Your dietary requirements could become a challenge if other aspects of the relationship are in flux or not as robust. As we discussed in chapters 4 through 6, some people are going to get on board right away, some will take a little time, and many will need some help, education, and patience, but most will be happy to support you.

Once you've discussed your options with your allergist and made a decision about what is best for your personal safety, have a conversation with your partner about how you would be most comfortable in your shared space. Here are some examples of topics to cover: the best course of action your allergist suggests, your feelings about your allergens generally and your feelings about your allergens near you, the needs of your partner (does he or she love peanut butter, but you're peanut-allergic and fearful?), the compromises you feel most comfortable with, and the best solution for now.

Remember, use "I" statements, talk about your needs in an open and gentle manner, keep your body language relaxed and flexible, and keep your facial muscles relaxed. If you feel yourself getting tense, reactive, or overly upset, take a step away from the topic, regain your composure, and return to the conversation when you feel more secure about your needs. Remember, your shared home should be a safe place for both people. Strive to create that space together.

emergency plans

Even the most vigilant of us can become complacent. Remember my kissing story with LT from the prologue? It wasn't until the next morning that I realized I didn't have any emergency plans in place anywhere in the apartment. All of my emergency information was in my head, except for what I had told LT. Being at home, I felt so comfortable that I overlooked this vital piece of information for guests and dates.

Immediately after this, I downloaded two plans, one for food allergies and one for asthma, from reliable sources. I filled them out with my pulmonologist (whom I saw the next day, because I was still wheezing) and posted them in my kitchen, where they remain. They are visual reminders of how a food allergy can progress, when to take what medication and how much, and emergency and medical contact numbers. Food-allergic reactions can happen anywhere and anytime, even in your safe haven, your home. Don't be caught unprepared. Not only should you know your emergency plan, you should make it public so others can know it, too.

where to get free downloadable food-allergy plans

- American Academy of Allergy Asthma and Immunology (AAAAI.org)
- American College of Allergy, Asthma, and Immunology (ACAAI.org)
- Anaphylaxis Canada (Anaphylaxis.ca)
- Asthma and Allergy Foundation of America (AAFA.org)
- Food Allergy Anaphylaxis Network (Foodallergy.org)
- Food Allergy Initiative (FAIUSA.org)

So—what are *your* rules about food allergies and your home? Do you keep your home completely scrubbed of every allergen? Do you allow foods to which you are allergic in your home? As you know from reading this chapter, I allow allergens to be brought into my home in a way that ensures my safety but allows my guests to not be restricted in their dining desires.

I came to that decision after many years of trying several variations. Too many allergens in my home was too scary; so that wasn't right. If no nuts were allowed, guests would forget or make mistakes and feel awful; that wasn't right either. I found a happy medium: allergens allowed, just not on my plates. (For how this works out on dates, see chapter 6.) As my confidence increased, I found a balance between safe and hospitable. That is the goal: safe for you, nice for company.

allergic girl's home safe home

- Home can be many different types of dwellings in different life stages; make a determination based on where you are right now.

- Can you, and do you, allow allergens to be brought into your home? This is the primary question.
- Confer with your medical Team You to help you make that determination.
- Talk with your Team You about the real risks involved with the level and severity of your food-allergic responses.
- Once you have verified what you need to do in order to stay safe, share the information verbally, in a nonconfrontational way, with those in your space.
- Even at home, mistakes can happen: cross-contamination of cooking utensils, processed foods, mislabeled ingredients, or just honest blunders.
- Go over your emergency plan with your allergist. Post a physical plan in common spaces, if applicable. Always have up-to-date medications on hand and know how and when to use them.

10

let's celebrate

One cannot have too large a party. A large
party secures its own amusement.

—Mr. Weston, *Emma* by Jane Austen

The invitation is stunning and sophisticated: white letters on a gray background. It's for the bar mitzvah of my cousin's son. It's still a few months away, so now is the perfect time to get in touch with the family about the kiddush (a light snack right after the ceremony) and the luncheon party menus. I sent a text to my cousin's wife: "Looking forward to your son's bar mitzvah. Don't want to make extra work for you, so am wondering if I may contact the caterer about the lunch menu. Let me know. Thanks!"

I received this reply: "Although we're looking forward to sharing this day with you, hopefully you can find something we're serving which satisfies your dietary needs." That would be a firm "No, you can't talk with the caterer. Just make do." Now what?

Whether you're going to a formal corporate work event or an informal baby shower, there are steps you can take to ensure that you get what you need during such celebrations and events, even if it means not eating at the event. Use the tips in this chapter in combination with the the primer concepts and the strategies we've already discussed for traveling, dining out, and dining in and you'll be able to join in the celebration whether dining (or not).

standard operating procedures

The following strategies constitute the standard operating procedures I teach, coach, and use to attend events successfully and join in the fun.

Communicate. E-mail the host, the event planner, the wedding coordinator, the caterer, or the chef. When your needs are written out, the possibility of playing the children's game telephone is greatly reduced (saying you have an "allergy to nuts" on the phone can turn into that person telling someone else that you "hate to make a fuss"). E-mail is therefore best here, because it can be referred to and passed around to other staff members. Tone is an essential component of the communication, especially since it can be misunderstood in writing. Keep your initial communication unmistakably polite, light, breezy, and positive. Send your communication as far in advance of the event as you can and follow up closer to the date.

Educate. You may need to educate extended family, hotel chefs, or caterers about what food allergies are, the danger of cross-contamination, and the easiest ways for you to stay safe. Keep it simple, clear, and to the point. Impart only vital information. Explain how an allergic reaction can manifest: itchy mouth, throat, eyes, or skin; hives; swelling or wheezing; or shock (anaphylaxis). Explain that you need your dishes prepared in an uncontaminated way. Suggest dishes that would work for you or offer to bring your own food if that is easiest. Stick to the facts of food allergies—two or three bullet points will suffice. This is not the time to start telling horror stories: "I almost died at the last wedding I attended" or "Aunt Bea tried to kill me by hiding walnuts in the turkey stuffing." Although these incidents are important to you, they can confuse the listener or frighten him or her unnecessarily.

Stay focused on the solution. While giving the list of what you can't eat, remember to give a list of what you *can* eat. Make a friendly, allergen-free suggestion. For formal events, I ask for a dry salad for starters, grilled or broiled meat or chicken with sautéed or steamed vegetables, and dry berries for dessert. Not only are these readily available in a hotel or a catering hall, they are free from the top eight allergens (eggs, milk, wheat, soy, peanuts, tree nuts, fish, and shellfish) and are inexpensive, healthy, and delicious. Create backup, safe menu alternatives to offer as suggestions.

Work within the system. Discuss how your needs can be accommodated within the existing menu or protocol. Make a personal determination to manage the risk and your expectations. If your extended family celebrates with a traditional Sicilian Christmas (fish dinner) and you're allergic to fish, then maybe bringing your own safe dish is the easiest solution. With some safe adjustments, however, if you can dine with the menu that is offered, go for it.

Be prepared. If you don't have the luxury of calling ahead of the event, don't panic. Go to the event prepared. Bring along a safe snack to munch on during the reception. Dine on something small before attending the event so you're not ravenously hungry. Focus on the purpose of the event rather than feeling left out because you're not dining on the rack of lamb in walnut pesto. If you're going out of your home area for the event, before you leave, have the name of a local hospital handy. Make sure you bring all of your medications and that they are up-to-date. Know where the local pharmacy is and bring the name of a local doctor, if possible. (See chapter 12 for more about traveling.)

find your sentence

How you describe your food-allergy needs to someone and what you actually disclose about those needs is a personal decision. My typical line is "I'm allergic to all tree nuts, fish, and shellfish." It's short and gets the point across. Of course, I've tried the complete truth with a server: "I'm allergic to tree nuts and salmon. I avoid all fish and shellfish according to my allergist's orders. I'm also allergic to eggplant and honeydew and cantaloupe melon but less severely. Sometimes tomatoes bother me and sometimes tropical fruits do but not always. " Understandably, that speech usually creates more confusion and anxiety for the server and the kitchen, which equals a more anxious Allergic Girl. So for now, "I'm allergic to all tree nuts, fish, and shellfish" is my go-to sentence, to start. I evaluate each menu and each situation individually and make adjustments accordingly to ensure the highest possibility of safety and clarity of my message.

In conjunction with your medical Team You, find a truthful sentence about your food-allergic needs that itemizes your dietary needs easily, gets the importance of your point across swiftly, and best ensures your safety in differing situations.

family and friends' events

Events, celebrations, and national or religious holidays are wonderful moments to be shared with loved ones. Following are some scenarios that illustrate the standard operating procedures in action.

The Thanksgiving Table

As we read in chapter 4, family members can be your biggest food-allergy allies. It was a week before Thanksgiving, and my cousin-in-law e-mailed me about the menu. We talked about what she was planning on making, what other people were bringing, and what I might need. I told her what I planned on eating (I don't need to have every dish), what I could contribute for the group, and what I would bring for myself. Here's a sample follow-up e-mail:

> Dear Lynn,
>
> Thank you again for taking the time to go over the menu with me. I really appreciate it! A gentle reminder: I'm allergic to all tree nuts, fish, and shellfish. Keeping the ingredients labels of anything you buy would really help; that way I can see exactly what's in everything without bugging you. What shall I bring? Dessert for everyone, side dishes, flowers for the table? Just let me know how I can make it easier for you while you're putting this together. Looking forward to seeing everyone.
>
> Much love,
>
> Cousin Sloane

When I arrived, Lynn walked me through the buffet, pointing out the one dish with pecans that was not for me and going through everything else. The meal is served buffet style, and I was first in line (fewer possibilities of cross-contamination). The one nutty dish was on a separate table—away from the turkey, cranberry sauce, and greens, which were the main things I wanted to eat. I took my portions and went back for second and third portions of the turkey and homemade cranberry sauce.

I had plenty of allies; my cousin's uncle is an allergist, and he and his wife brought the turkey. I trust Lynn; she's always been sensitive to my needs and is a terrific hostess. She knows about cross-contamination because there are many children in her daughters' school with food allergies, and the mothers have been instructed about how to send treats to school. I had my medications on me, and I had my meal plan; that is, I knew what I was going to be eating, and I knew what on the menu was off-limits because Lynn and I had discussed it beforehand. Can it be this easy? Yes, it can.

Bringing Your Own

As we also read in chapter 4, sometimes it's family that can be the most rigid and least understanding about your needs. Starting when I was sixteen years old (and for seventeen years thereafter), I maintained an ovo-lacto vegetarian diet of eggs, dairy, legumes, vegetables, and grains. In addition to having food allergies, I voluntarily chose not to eat any meat.

During those years, when a different cousin-in-law hosted family holidays, I brought a safe veggie dish from home. With this branch of the family, I knew it was easier to say, "Don't worry about my dinner, I'll take care of it." I didn't discuss the menu with the hostess, discuss potential safe side dishes or issues of cross-contamination, educate them about my choice to be vegetarian, or try to fit in with the planned menu. Managing expectations seemed to be the best course of action.

Even though I tried to avoid problems by bringing my own food, there were still nonverbal (and some verbal) harrumphs from this cousin, who wanted to know why I couldn't just eat what she was serving. I shrugged it off with a laugh, happily digging into my safe veggie dinner, and rapidly changed the topic. (Go back to chapter 4 for suggestions on how to handle family members who don't understand your needs.)

Back to the opening scenario of this chapter, the bar mitzvah: This is the same branch of the family that was not pleased when I brought my own food for Thanksgiving. Even though it's been some years since these relatives hosted Thanksgiving, my hunch was that I would probably not be welcomed at the bar mitzvah with open, allergen-free arms. I made a concerted effort to reach out with a friendly and gentle communication—a "let me make this easy for you" message—but I received a very clear no-go. I had a choice: register this wrong and rant to any family member who would listen or bring my own food and join in the fun. I chose the latter.

Bringing your own food, whether to a family event, a corporate event, or a wedding, is always an option. It's a fail-safe, it eliminates multiple concerns, the control is completely with you, and you can focus on the event.

Tonight We'll Be Dining on Lamb

Rosh Hashanah, the Jewish New Year, is one of my favorite holidays, not merely because it's in the fall, which I love, and it's a time for inner reflection, which I also love, but also because the food is *so* divine. The last few years, my dear and safe friend Stéphanie has invited my family to join hers to celebrate.

Stéphanie's traditions are Sephardic; mine are Ashkenazi. The foods of Sephardic Jews have a Spanish, Mediterranean, and North African influence; the foods of Ashkenazi Jews have an eastern European influence. When Americans think about typical Jewish food, they are usually thinking about Ashkenazi cuisine: matzo ball soup, brisket, knishes, and bagels. Sephardic food uses spices traditional to the Mediterranean and the Middle East, such as cumin, cinnamon, a greater variety of beans and grains (even during Passover, when Ashkenazi Jews don't eat beans or rice in addition to breads and pastas), and lamb as well as beef.

Stéphanie makes a lamb and prune dish that drives me bonkers with happiness. One year, the holiday guest list was a potential hostess nightmare: me with my allergies; my mother, who has different food allergies from me; a vegetarian who is gluten-intolerant; and a friend who eats no vegetables or fruit (by preference). It was a lot for a hostess to juggle, but Stéphanie was up to the task. She makes everything from scratch, so she knows her ingredients inside and out. To make it easier for everyone, she introduced each dish with a list of its ingredients as a special nod to everyone's needs, so we all knew exactly what we could eat and what we could not.

Prior to the holiday, I sent an e-mail with a gentle reminder of my needs and asking what I could do to help:

Dear Stéphanie,

I can't wait for Rosh with your family. Thank you again for your kind invitation. I'm so looking forward to it. Just a gentle reminder, I'm allergic to tree nuts, fish, and shellfish. You know I can't wait for the famous lamb dish; can we go over its ingredients again? What shall I bring? If you need help, I'm happy to come early to assist with setup or stay late for clean-up duty; just let me know.

Much love,

Sloane

Stéphanie is a special friend, undoubtedly. She's an excellent chef; she respects her ingredients as well as the needs of her guests. Dining with her family is always a pleasure, on both a personal and a culinary level, and safe.

formal events

Formal events—like weddings, engagements, and religious celebrations (like bar mitzvahs)— that take place in a hotel, a restaurant, or a catering hall can be simpler than home-based events because there is usually a catering manager or a general manager who will handle your requests. Hotels in particular are used to dealing with special requests.

If you can, give the catering director notice before the event you're attending; a phone call placed early to let him or her know what you would like, with lots of pleases and thank-yous, can do wonders. You can sidestep family drama and make it worry-free for everyone (yourself, foremost) by dealing directly with the caterers.

If you are asking for something off-menu or for a specialty item, offer to take care of any extra costs. When you talk with the caterers, tell them to deal with you directly about any additional charges. The idea is to make this effortless, not cost-prohibitive, for the host, the event planner, the bride, or the birthday boy. If it's more cost-effective for you to bring your own dish and have the caterers warm it up or keep it cool, ask them about that, too.

A Member of the Wedding

Isabel is a dear, safe friend whom I've known for more than fifteen years. When she was married recently, I was her witness in the signing of the *ketubah* (the Jewish marriage contract), and I was one of the speakers during the ceremony. Isabel put me in touch with the caterer directly a week before the event—the wedding was at a restaurant, but she used an outside catering company. Her e-mail to her caterers, which she copied me on, was as follows:

> Dear Robert,
>
> Remember that I mentioned a while back that there would be one special meal? Well, the special meal is for my dearest friend, Sloane, who is sitting at my table. I would like you two to talk directly to make sure Sloane isn't allergic to anything in her dinner. She also may require a different first course. Take it from here, you two!
>
> Best,
>
> Isabel

Here is my follow-up e-mail to the caterer:

> Good morning, Robert!
>
> Thank you in advance for taking care of this. I have some food allergies and food intolerances that I'd like to make you aware of. I'm allergic to all tree nuts, fish, and shellfish. It's probably easier to discuss particulars over

the phone about your menu and how we can make this easy for everyone. Thank you!

Best,

Sloane

I followed up with a phone call later that day, and the chef of the catering group and I went over the menu of what was going to be served and what adjustments would work for my needs. We settled on a dry salad for starters, short ribs and vegetables, and berries for dessert.

When I arrived at the reception, I found the chef in the restaurant kitchen and introduced myself. She said, "We brought your meal in a completely separate container." I had eaten a late lunch so I wouldn't be hungry through the ceremony and the beginning of the reception with the passed hors d'oeuvres, which the chef had told me were off-limits to me (all fish). When we sat down my food was on plates of a color different from all the others, making it very easy to identify. After the meal, I made a quick trip to the kitchen to thank the catering staff. While there I also spied a cooler labeled with big black letters: Food Allergy Plate. A few days after the wedding I sent e-mails to thank the caterer and the bride for taking care of me.

Avoiding the Raw Bar

The morning of my friend Allison's wedding, I called the hotel and asked for the catering department. I had not spoken to the bride about my needs but had bypassed the wedding party entirely. (This doesn't work for every allergic guest or for every wedding party, but I knew Allison would appreciate my taking care of this during her busy time. Your goal is to have a direct conversation with the catering staff, not to play telephone. Do whatever works best.)

I spoke with the catering manager, and gave him my spiel: I'm allergic to tree nuts, fish, and shellfish. He told me the wedding menu: salmon and caviar, to start; the choice of rack of lamb or sea bass for the main course, and chocolate with nuts for dessert. It was an excellent menu, to be sure, but not one in which I could indulge.

The smart manager then asked me, "What would you like us to make for you?" I gave him my usual safe-event menu: dry green salad, broiled chicken with steamed mixed veggies, and berries for dessert. He said, "We can do that easily." As extra insurance, I ate something at home before I went so that I wouldn't be really hungry during the after-ceremony appetizers. I'm glad I did, because the focus at this extravagant wedding was an open raw bar and shellfish station. I opted for champagne and steered clear of the cracking king crab legs mosh pit.

Once we were seated, I introduced myself to my table's server and said that I had spoken to the manager. The server confirmed that he was aware of me and my needs. I reiterated my allergies with many pleases and thank-yous and smiled a lot. It was all pretty darn easy, and I could fully concentrate on getting my wedding groove on. When the bride and the groom came by our table for a picture, Allison leaned in and asked me if I had found something to eat. "Yes, they did a great job," I replied.

Catered Birthdays

Recently my cousin Gregg had a milestone-birthday party. Invited were a combination of his friends and the immediate family. It was at a country club golf course in Connecticut on a lovely summer day—that is, a place with a big catering kitchen. I hadn't realized that it was a catered event, or I would have called earlier. So I did many of the steps that I use when dining out with complete success.

When I arrived, I asked for the catering manager. I introduced myself, and she introduced herself. I complimented her dress, smiled, and told her about my needs. The buffet was completely out (fish, chicken in a nutty sauce, salad with contaminated tongs—nothing safe), so I asked if she might be able to make me some plain broiled chicken with just vegetable oil and salt and pepper and steamed green veggies. She said, "Absolutely no problem. Where are you sitting?" Within moments of our discussion, exactly what we had discussed arrived. Surmising that I couldn't have dessert, the catering manager took the initiative and brought out a plate of fresh berries. How lovely and simple is that?

work events

Work events have an added pressure of being with work colleagues and bosses while eating and drinking. Don't let that pressure supplant you getting what you need food-allergy-wise and joining in. All of the strategies we've explored so far work well here, too. Read the following scenarios to get a feel for how these strageties look in action.

Holiday Parties

My last corporate job was with a midsized, foreign-owned, multi-state operation. When it was time for the first corporate Christmas party, I felt too shy to ask about what was being served. At the time I was still an ovo-lacto vegetarian as well as food-allergic. The menu was saucy ribs, pork and beans, dressed salad with walnuts, macaroni and cheese with ham, and collard greens with bacon; there was not one thing I could eat. So, I had a drink, stayed for the toasts, and slunk away early. I did none of the allergy-safe food steps, missed all of the fun, and lost out on the holiday sucking-up-to-the-boss time.

The next year, the party was at a seafood restaurant nearby. My gut reaction was "Oh, no! What am I going to do—a whole night of fish, and it's the Christmas party!" I had a moment of thinking that maybe I should just skip it. That thought was quickly vanquished as I became determined to find a way to make it safe and fun; I didn't want to miss out for a second year because of food allergies.

Since the company had offices across the country, different departments were all over; half of the people with whom I worked I had never met. Through some calling around and asking some higher-ups, I discovered that the New York vice president of sales was doing most of the planning. Just as I was poised to send her my standard e-mail (I have some food allergies, what's the menu, whom can I talk to about adjustments), my direct boss said she knew the owner and chef of the restaurant. She put me in touch with him directly.

I did a version of the dining-out steps (see chapter 11). The chef-owner and I had a lengthy conversation about my needs; we talked about the menu and what adjustments could be made easily and safely. He seemed very knowledgeable about food allergies and cross-contamination issues. As a restaurant owner and chef for more than twenty years, he was culinarily experienced and welcoming. He said he would take care of me personally and that I should identify myself when I got to the restaurant.

Because the restaurant specialized in fish, I still brought a safe snack, just in case I didn't feel so safe once I was on-site. But when I arrived and introduced myself to the chef, he assured me that everyone was ready for me. Everything that was served to me was indeed fish- and nut-free.

A Catered Work Event On-Site

I was speaking on a blogging panel for a conference at a university club in Midtown Manhattan. There was a luncheon as part of the day's activities for a few hundred of us. Because I was speaking, the last thing I wanted to be focused on was any dining difficulties; I wanted to be as relaxed and focused as possible. So I ate something before I went, I brought snacks with me, and I did a version of the standard operating procedure.

Once on-site at lunch, just before my panel, my special meal request was nowhere to be found. They had lost the request and the special meal. In a flash, the young floor manager came over and asked what I'd like for lunch. Since I had noshed beforehand, just in case of an occurrence like this, I asked for some plain fruit. He offered a starter of a berry plate. Everyone at the table stopped talking and looked at me as my gorgeous berry plate arrived.

"How did you get that?" asked my clearly envious tablemates.

"Food allergies," I said with a big smile, which sparked an interesting discussion. The berries were plentiful, so I shared them with my tablemates. I was impressed with how quickly the kitchen management was able to get me something yummy to eat in a room full of two hundred food publicists and marketers. I also didn't leave much to chance, however, since I had eaten beforehand and packed some snacks. Being prepared, especially for an important meeting, takes the pressure off—one less thing to worry about.

A Catered Work Event with an Outside Vendor

Recently I was asked to participate on a different panel discussion, this time for women in social media. A week before the event, the organizer e-mailed the panelists with what to prepare for our conversation and other details. The panel was going to be held during lunchtime, so lunch was going to be served. Again I used my standard operating procedures to see what accommodations could be made and determine what would be both easiest for me and for the group. I responded to that e-mail with "What are they serving for lunch, so I may coordinate my dietary needs?" Immediately the panel producer wrote back and copied the event organizer.

I followed up directly:

Dear Rose,

I'm allergic to all nuts and fish. If it would be easier to chat, I can be reached at the number below. Looking forward.

Best, Sloane

The organizer wrote back:

> Hi Sloane,
>
> Our host is assisting with the selection of a nearby deli.
> The luncheon will be a sandwich buffet. So she definitely
> will need to talk with you about your diet restrictions.
>
> Rose

I called right away and gave her a list of what would be ideal and
also offered to bring my own lunch if that was simpler. Again,
since this was a work function and I was the speaker, the last thing
I wanted to be concerned with was the food. I followed up the
phone exchange with a clear e-mail that could be easily forwarded
to the food purveyor:

> It was lovely speaking with you just now, Rose. As we
> discussed, the simpler the better, as I'm allergic to all
> tree nuts, fish, and shellfish. Here are some easy options.
> Sliced cheese like Muenster, jack, or provolone. Sliced
> deli meats like turkey. And fruit like strawberries. All
> plain, without sauce or garnish. Thank you and I'm
> available to discuss at any time.

When I arrived at the event, I was greeted by Rose, who had my
special brown bag lunch at her seat: sliced turkey, sliced cheese,
and berries. All plain, all fine. Again, I had snacks with me and
had eaten just before, as insurance. But by the time the panel concluded, it was an hour and half later and I was hungry. With just
a few friendly, clear e-mails, and even having to deal with multiple
people, it was easy to get my food-allergic needs met.

go celebrate!

Don't think for one minute that you have to miss out on holidays,
family or friends' celebrations, life-cycle events, or work-related

events just because you can't eat Aunt Bea's special nut-studded Jell-O mold or share the boss's pupu platter. Reach out to the person in charge, make an assessment about his or her ability to serve something you can consume safely, and go, go, go!

allergic girl's party-time tips

- Communicate, educate, be solution-oriented, work within the menu, and be prepared. These basic steps, coupled with the primer concepts will enable you to go to any event anywhere and ensure your safety.
- A sense of humor will keep you sane. Use it. Do your best to laugh off miscommunications, misunderstandings, or any meanness.
- Review the zigzag technique (see chapter 4) for dealing with those who don't get it.
- Have backup plans: having your medications on you at all times, eating before you go, taking safe snacks in your purse or bag, and asking for an ideal safe menu item that most hotels or catering halls would have on hand (whether you talk to the catering manager beforehand or on-site).
- Focus is crucial here. Once you have ensured your personal safety, focus on the purpose of the event, whether it's a national holiday, a religious event, a work event, or a family day.

11

read the restaurant

Sally is a great orderer. Not only does she always pick
the best thing in the menu, but she orders it in a way
that the chef didn't even know how good it could be.

—Harry Burns, *When Harry Met Sally*

I was meeting my friends Josh and Mauro for dinner at a
Lebanese restaurant in the Flatiron District. Earlier that day, I
had spoken with the general manager and asked her if the chef felt
comfortable handling food allergies. She said that he did. "We will
take great care of you," she added.

When I arrived at the restaurant (a little earlier than the group,
in order to talk with the manager about my needs), I identified
myself at the host's station.

"Hi, I'm Sloane. I'm here for a seven-thirty reservation. I called
earlier and spoke with the manager about my food allergies. Is she
available?"

"Oh, yes, of course. Hi. Welcome. We're happy to have you. The chef created a special menu for you. It's all printed out, and when you're seated your server will bring it to you. Let us know if there's anything else we can do. As soon as your party is here, we will seat you." The general manager explained that the special menu had no tree nuts, fish, or shellfish.

Josh was already at the bar. We hugged and chatted, and when Mauro arrived, we all sat down. When we chose our seats, our server put down all of the menus and, for me, there was a printed one that was labeled "Sloane's menu." Inside was an abbreviated version of the larger menu, containing only items that were identified as Sloane-friendly, taken from the list I had given the restaurant earlier that day. Our server proceeded to take everyone's order and then came around to me.

"Hi, I'm Sloane. So is this chicken really just garlic and lemon?"

"Hi. I'm Dave," he said, "and yes, it is. It's totally safe for you."

"Great, I'd love the chicken, and could I get the salad but with no sumac dressing?"

"Sure."

"Just to remind you, I'm allergic to nuts, fish, and shellfish. I know they told you, but I just wanted to double check. Thank you for taking care of my needs, it's really appreciated."

"Of course," Dave said, "If you need anything or have any further questions, I'm here."

As every dish was placed in front of me, it was identified as nut-, fish-, and shellfish-free by the food runner (a person who brings the food but is not your server). Josh asked me if I wanted to try some of the mini lamb sausages. I said that I'd better not, since they weren't on my special menu and I didn't know what was in them. A food runner overheard us talking and said, "Don't eat those; they have pine nuts in them." Freshly baked pita (with a nut spread) was brought to the table, and a runner presented me with complimentary vegetable crudités. Mauro asked, "Where's this extra food coming from?" I jokingly said, "Didn't you know, people with food allergies are the new VIPs." The next day I e-mailed the owner and chef, thanking him for providing excellent service and taking care of me. He replied immediately, with graciousness and appreciation.

Is this real or a dream? Only in a dream, you might think, could people with food allergies ever get this kind of treatment—unless they know the owner, tip everyone in hundred-dollar bills, or demand that everyone take care of their allergy needs or prepare to be sued. I didn't know the owner, I don't walk around with crisp hundreds for whoever will make me something allergen-free (I wish), and I never threaten a restaurant's staff.

I dine out at least five nights a week and at one new restaurant a week, at minimum. I rely on time-tested quantifiable techniques that have given scores of food-allergy coaching clients consistent and safe results. I even created a highly successful exclusive food-allergy dining membership group called Worry-Free Dinners based on these transferable techniques. I'm going to present a typical allergen-friendly dining-out occurrence, break it down into the requirements for a positive experience, and point out if and when you should cut your losses.

Before you go out anywhere, you need to know what you are going to say to that all-important manager, chef, owner or server to get the food allergy ball rolling. As we explored in chapter 10, it's vital that you have one truthful sentence about your food allergy needs that gets your point across swiftly and clearly. Often, when dining out, especially at a busy restaurant, there's only a small window of opportunity in which to grab someone's attention and let him or her know about your dietary restrictions and their severity. That's why you need a sentence or two that does all the work in a short amount of time.

three top new york city–based restaurant groups that partner with worry-free dinners

B. R. Guest restaurants, www.brguestrestaurants.com
Craft Restaurants, www.craftrestaurant.com
Union Square Hospitality Group, www.ushgnyc.com

So, in conjunction with your medical Team You, safe person or food allergy coach, create that one (or two) sentence about your food allergic needs that you can use to impart your vital information. This sentence, or statement, should itemize your dietary needs easily, get the importance of your point across swiftly, which will ensure your safety and minimize risk. (Read more in the chapter to see my statement in action.) Remember that you want to start a dialogue with a restaurant, so keep the tone light, no demands or threats, and clear and firm. If you feel like you might freeze up the first time you use your statement, practice it with a safe friend or in the mirror; write it down on a business card or copy it down in your smart phone. Above all, find your "I'm allergic to . . ." statement and use it.

read the table

In restaurant-speak, servers are supposed to "read" the table. This means that they are supposed to get a sense of what the table needs and provide it appropriately. In many dining establishments, the servers are salespeople: selling you an extra appetizer, a dessert, the bigger-ticket items, or drinks. So, in theory, a server should do his or her best to read what the table wants and can afford.

Is this a liquid-lunch business meeting? In that case, the server will be by every ten minutes or so to take additional drink orders. Is this a date? Then perhaps the couple would like a chocolaty dessert to share. Are these ladies from out of town on a shopping spree? Perhaps they need some assistance about where to go next, along with another round of watermelon daiquiris. If a diner is scraping the sauce off the chicken or pushing unwanted food around the plate, the server should inquire why. Was something wrong with the dish? Is there a food-allergy issue or concern? The server should be reading you, your needs, and the table's needs.

For the food-allergic diner who wants to dine out as safely as possible, your job is to read the restaurant from the instant you check out its Web site, to calling ahead, to the minute you step over the threshold and place an order. At every moment of your encounter, you will receive essential information about how your needs will be accommodated. I'm going to break down these micromoments to see what information can be garnered where and when, and how to make safe decisions accordingly.

vet the menu

The first step, when you want to dine out, is to do some research on the restaurant. Go to the restaurant's Web site and look at the menu. If there are dishes or ingredients you've never heard of, Google them. In three clicks or less, you can find out that Mexican mole sauce typically contains ground peanuts and/or tree nuts or that Thai cuisine uses a fish sauce base in most dishes. You can rule out certain dishes based on your particular needs and manage your risk before you even walk through the door.

Does the restaurant menu online say in fine print on the bottom, "No substitutions"? That will give you some insight into the restaurant's philosophy. Or does the menu's fine print say, "Let your server know about allergies or any dietary restrictions"? That gives you a clue that the restaurant will be amenable to your requests.

Is there something on the menu that you would like or that seems as though it could be altered relatively easily, such as a protein without a sauce or a mixed salad without dressing? Don't go to a restaurant if there's nothing on the menu you'd like to eat. Again, it may seem like a simple step, but it will save you so much aggrevation to know what you might like when walking in the door. With dietary restrictions, it's rare that an entire menu will be available to you. So find up to three dishes that would be of interest to you and have them in mind when you go.

Read the "About Us" section of the restaurant's Web site as well as the chef's philosophy. Chef Mark Zeitouni of the Standard Spa in Miami Beach says, "A diner should first understand the delineation between going to a restaurant that is a vehicle for a star chef versus a restaurant that caters to the diner. A star chef will serve you what he or she wants. It will probably be outstanding, but for a diner with specific needs, it will not necessarily be what you need. Pick a place that caters to the diner, not the other way around."

Look for a restaurant that focuses on its patrons, using phrases such as these: "We redefine the restaurant experience with an emphasis on hospitality, style, and accessible cuisine" or "Each of our restaurants strives to distinguish itself for its unparalleled cuisine and warm hospitality." Attention to customers and focus on hospitality—that's what you're looking for.

Here's a sample e-mail exchange between me and a restaurant I had been to once before. It had been able to make modifications to the menu on the spot, so this time I looked over the dinner menu online, isolated two items that if not allergen-free at least looked easy to modify, and e-mailed the manager two days ahead of our proposed dinner.

Hi,

I hope this e-mail finds you very well! I had such a nice experience last time with you and your team that we were thinking of coming to an early dinner Thursday night. I took a look at the menu online and was thinking maybe the duck or the lamb would be possible with my allergies. A reminder: I'm allergic to all tree nuts, fish, and shellfish. Let me know your thoughts.

Thank you and best wishes,

Sloane

This was the manager's reply:

Hi, Sloane,

This is the word from the chef: Lamb, yes. Duck, yes.
We look forward to having you join us on Thursday. Let
me know when you'd like a reservation, and we will see
you then.

The e-mail was straightforward and simple; the dinner delicious
and safe. The chef even joined us tableside for a chat and to check
in on our meal. Vet the menu and start the communication as
early as possible.

call ahead

Call the restaurant before you go and ask to speak with the manager or the chef about your allergies and the restaurant's ability to
deal with them. It's best to call in between shifts (before lunch or
after; before dinner or after) when the manger will be less busy and
can focus on your requests. If the person who answers the phone
is a host and seems confused about what food allergies are, remain
calm but make a mental note that the restaurant might not have
a well-trained front-of-house staff. If the person who answers the
phone tells you that the manager or the chef is too busy, that's
information, too. When you finally do speak to the manager, ask
his or her name and give yours; create some phone rapport. Repeat
your request. If the manager says they can handle your request
with ease, then go, but remain cautious.

A Direct Line to the Chef

I was running low on time, so I once called a restaurant only hours
before our eight-thirty reservation. When I mentioned that I had
food allergies, the reservationist said, "Let me put you through
to the kitchen to talk with them directly." I spoke with the chef,
who said, "We can handle all of your allergies. We can easily make

substitutions, it won't be a problem." That's what you want: a direct line to the kitchen.

A Direct Line to Nowhere

My safe friend Shari suggested we try somewhere new for dinner one Friday night, an authentic ethnic restaurant. I looked at the menu online; there were lots of nutty, fishy things, but also some nonnutty, nonfishy dishes. I called ahead and spoke with the hostess, who gave me all the information I needed to determine that this was not the restaurant for me.

"Hi. I'm thinking of coming in to dine tonight, and I'm allergic to tree nuts, fish, and shellfish. I'm wondering if the kitchen feels comfortable handling that."

"So, you're a vegan?"

"No, I'm not a vegan; I'd happily eat meat. I'm severely allergic to foods. Tree nuts, fish, and shellfish will make me very ill if I consume them accidentally."

"So you don't eat tuna fish or tree-what?"

This telephone exchange indicated that there was a miscommunication, at least, and at most, we were going nowhere, fast. Whoever picks up the phone will give you an indication of your evening. There are exceptions, of course. But there's nothing wrong with trusting your gut based on who answers the phone. Shari and I ate elsewhere.

online reservations

Another new tool for diners with special requests is an online reservation system. These are services that send your reservation and your request to the restaurant, or you can often book directly through the restaurant's site. Write a short note:

Dear Manager,

I'm looking forward to dining at your restaurant this evening. Please note: I'm severely allergic to tree nuts, fish, and shellfish. Thank you for your kind attention to this matter.

Best wishes, Sloane

Using an online system also cuts out the telephone game of talking to a host or hostess; your needs are spelled out clearly for everyone to see. You have to register to use the service, so it has your e-mail address and phone number in order to check with you if there is an issue. The use of these systems automatically tips off restaurant managers to enact their allergen protocols (if they have them). My experience using these systems and recommending them for my clients is that once you trigger their allergen protocol though the online system, a manager will greet you and confirm the allergy; the chef, the server, and the food runners are aware; and everyone checks with you again along the way. It's fantastic.

For a recent date, Dan and I went to a restaurant at which he had made reservations using a national online reservation system. Dan e-mailed all of my allergies ahead of time. When we arrived, the manager was prepared for us, the server had my allergies all nicely typed out, and we were told that the chef had been informed of my needs and was happy to make adjustments to any item on the menu. They were totally ready for me, and they seemed happy to see us, which is always a big plus. Dan and I even shared some dishes. Bites were passed, tastes were savored, dinner was yummy; it was a great date. And it all started by using an online reservation system to list my allergies.

chef cards

When you're dining either at home or on the road, chef cards are a great help. These are preprinted cards you take along with you that list your allergens and may even have a picture of the forbidden

free or low-cost chef cards

Allergy Translation, https://allergytranslation.com
Culinary Institute of America, www.ciaprochef.com/
    foodallergies/about.html
Food Allergy and Anaphylaxis Network, www.Foodallergy
    .org
Food Allergy Initiative, www.faiusa.org
Select Wisely, www.Selectwisely.com

ingredient as well. They are usually laminated or on coated paper, which makes them very durable. Cards are available in multiple languages, so they are great for traveling abroad or eating in ethnic restaurants. I've spoken to scores of chefs, and they love chef cards, because this tool, like many we've explored, eliminates confusion or playing the telephone game. Having your allergens spelled out in black white (or red) is an excellent tool; use it.

when to dine

If you can, make a reservation for an early meal on a less busy day. These details are not always in your control, but when they are, use them. Dining early in the evening and on a less busy day will increase the chance that you will have an allergen-friendly meal with fewer issues. (Monday, Tuesday, and Wednesday are typically less busy, but when you call ahead, you can ask the manager that as well.) Making a reservation for eight-thirty on a Saturday night at a restaurant you've never been to before increases the risk of problems or complications with your order. It's a simple fact that when the kitchen staff is busier, it will be less able to concentrate on you. There may be plenty of restaurants that can handle your request on a busy Saturday, but as of this writing, there are far more that can't.

on-site

When you arrive, ask for the manager or the chef (by name, if you've called ahead). Present a chef card or give the manager a verbal list of the foods to avoid. Make sure the person writes down your list. Go over the menu and discuss your options—even before you get to the table, if you can. Standing up while you have this conversation, seeing the other person eye to eye, works better on so many levels.

Reconfirm Your Needs

When you sit down, reconfirm with your server that you talked with the manager. Tell the server what your allergies are, even if he or she has already been informed. It's no one's else's job but yours to memorize your needs. If you have to verbally confirm your needs with the server after every course, do it. Smile and be nice, but be firm about what your needs are. (Remember the story in chapter 5 about the scallop sauce dripping into my chicken dish. Back it went, despite the server's resistance.)

Some servers won't write down your allergies or your order. Be incredibly wary. An article in the *Washington Post* (January 12, 2010) looked at the old-school serving style in which the server rattles off the whole menu and takes your order without writing down a thing. The *Post* admitted that because of the way diners eat now, memorizing a table's order is not as practical or as elegant as it once may have been. Thank goodness. For those of us with dietary restrictions, it's imperative that a server does not try to memorize them. I can't say it enough: It's your job to memorize your allergies—not the server's. So if a server isn't writing down your order, I suggest that you kindly request that he or she do so. Smile and say it nicely, not in a demanding way, but make sure that your needs are written down. You can always use a chef card, where it's already all written out.

Tip Well

If all goes well, tip well. If there is a feedback card, fill it out. Write down the names of whoever helped you: the server, the manger, and the chef. The comments will go in their files, and it will help the restaurant to know what an allergic diner needs. The comments will also flag you for next time (in a good way), and the restaurant staff will get to know you and your needs better. It's part of becoming a regular, and that's what you want to be.

send a thank-you note

If applicable, make a phone call, send a card or an e-mail thank-you note the next day; it is always appreciated. It reinforces that you are a potentially good and loyal customer, that the allergen protocol the restaurant has in place works, and that the staff should keep up the good work.

Simple works best here. After the dinner with my friends Josh and Mauro, I sent a note to the chef the next day. (His e-mail address was on the Web site.) It was simple, straightforward, and well received:

> Dear Chef,
>
> I was the food-allergic guest last night. Dave took excellent care of me, and the personalized printed menu was great. I will return, and I look forward to trying more of your menu, especially the lamb. Thank you again.
>
> Very best wishes,
>
> Sloane

The chef replied:

> Thank you for the kind words. Just so that you know, we have a no "no" policy at the restaurant. We simply

will do everything we can to accommodate any request possible.

Kind regards,

Chef

Easy, right? And the way is paved for the next visit.

the bad, the rude, and the salvagable

If you've had food allergies for any length of time, I bet you've had a negative experience with a restaurant. Following are some examples of negative restaurant experiences and practical strategies for how to manage your food-allergy risk, deal with rude waitstaff, and even salvage a restaurant experience from the brink of bad to excellent and fun. (Yes, it can be done.)

Deciding When to Leave without Eating

I was on a second date at a fancy restaurant that I knew very well and trusted. We sat at the bar, and the bartender wasn't paying attention; he was curt and unfriendly, and I was getting a bad feeling that not only was I not being heard, I also wouldn't be able to enjoy my date or my meal. So I turned to my date told him that I felt uncomfortable. He suggested that we leave.

Chef Franklin Becker of Abe and Arthur's in New York City once told me, "If you go to a restaurant and that's the feeling the owners and/or the staff give you, you should get up and go someplace else, because they don't deserve your business. If that's their reaction to you, the odds are that your needs are not being communicated to the chef correctly, and there's a good chance you are playing Russian roulette with your health at that restaurant."

Sometimes it's easiest to just cut your losses and leave. If you feel bashful that you're leaving a restaurant before you've eaten (or even ordered), remember that no one's really looking. Staying in a situation that you think is already doomed doesn't help anyone. It's a strength to know when to bow out of a potentially dangerous dining situation.

The Server Zigzag

The eye roll, the pity look, the head shake, the tsk-tsk, and comments like "Oh my gosh, what do you eat?", "Jeez, how do you live?" or "Ugh, how horrible" are very common server editorials on food allergies. We've all experienced these reactions, but they're particularly disconcerting when you're on a date, at a work dinner, or all dressed up and with friends at a hot new restaurant.

Whenever possible, have the food-allergy conversation about your needs away from the table and your group, meeting, or date. If you've spoken to the manager or the staff ahead of time the odds are that the server will be well-informed of your needs and that those comments won't happen tableside. If you didn't have time to do that step, however, don't panic.

Instead, preempt. Once everyone sits down in your group, excuse yourself, find the manager or server for your table, and discuss your needs away from the table. Remember to employ a relaxed posture, be friendly, create some rapport, introduce yourself by name, and be assertive. Explain what your needs are and go over the menu together, again away from your group. If you can't find your server or feel shy about leaving your group to talk one-to-one with the manager or the server, go ahead and have the conversation at the table.

However, if your server weighs in negatively and publicly about your food allergies, remember the zigzag technique; it works very well here, too. Example: "Oh my gosh, what do you eat?" Reply: "I eat everything, just not tree nuts, fish, or shellfish, so if you could check with the chef that those things aren't in my meal, that would be great." Stay polite and take the higher ground; whatever you do, do not get into a skirmish at the table. It's not worth the trouble. (If you've done this once, you'll understand why.)

Downright Rude Comments

"Wow. I wouldn't want to be you." Chances are you've heard some variation of this, or worse, when telling a chef, a manager, or a server about your dietary restrictions and needs. Comments of this nature from any type of service-industry employee should be reported to management. These statements should never happen between a server and a patron (or a hotel worker and a guest or a caterer and a guest). This indicates a lack of training of the part of management, not only about food allergies but also about patron relations and hospitality.

Make sure you know the name of your server so you can refer to him or her by name, and make sure to talk to the manager before you leave the restaurant. If you feel shy about confronting the manager on-site, send an e-mail or call *the next day* to make sure that the management knows how its restaurant is being represented. If you wait too long, the details will be obscured, the server's and manager's shifts will have changed, and the staff will be different. If you're going to send an e-mail, do it within twenty-four hours, after you've calmed down but when everyone is still there. Keep your e-mail simple and to the point:

Dear Manager,

I dined at your establishment last evening. Upon telling our server, Adam, that I had food allergies and asking about your menu, he replied, "I wouldn't want to be you." This was disconcerting to hear. Your establishment came highly recommended, and I was deeply dismayed by this server's comment. I thought you would want to know.

Sincerely,

Sloane Miller

These kinds of comments and this kind of behavior is unacceptable, and any restaurant that cares about its patrons would want to know so that it can correct it.

When You Can't Leave

You're out with your new boss. You're with a large raucous party. You're at a family event. You're on a hot date. You're meeting your buddies, and it was hard enough just agreeing on a place and time. You've done all of the steps and used the primer concepts, and your food allergy requests are still being met with resistance, a brick wall, eye rolls, and a lack of comprehension. You're trying to stay upbeat, but you have a sinking feeling that this is going to go horribly wrong. Worst of all, you're committed to this event; you cannot leave. Ideally, you're prepared with a snack or you ate a little something beforehand, so you're not incredibly hungry. But life is often not ideal. So, you still have several options.

Have a go-to backup dish or meal that you know most restaurants have and is safe for you. When all else fails, one of my go-to meals is a baked potato with steamed broccoli and melted cheese. Potatoes are baked solo, usually earlier in the day, so that's pretty safe. Steamed broccoli can be made easily, and melted cheese is simple. Any restaurant should have all of these items on hand, and they are not normally near any nutty and fishy things. I don't require an ally or good enough trust to order this meal and be safe. Now think about some go-to options for yourself.

Find a temporary safe person in your group. It is possible that you've gotten so worked up about not being able to dine that you've got "the face" on (indignant, angry, annoyed, stressed, self-righteous) and are seeing nonallies everywhere. Make a safe friend on the spot and ask him or her to help you get you needs met. Maybe a more detached person can ask the server some questions without getting the eye roll. Sometimes when you're too close to it, when it's too important, you can see allergy enemies everywhere. An instant safe person can assist you with cutting through the anxiety and getting a server to help you.

Go deeper to find a restaurant ally. Stay calm and envision the type of person who will understand. Excuse yourself and ask to see another general manager. Ask to see the executive chef or the owner. Be firm, be assertive—find the one manager or server in the restaurant who understands enough to ensure that you can get something safe. If you do a little bit more digging, sometimes you'll find that the person with attitude was just an exception.

If you're feeling shy with the people you're with because you don't really know anyone and there's not an ally to be found, don't panic. However, do *not* eat. It's not worth the risk. Excuse yourself and make a run to the nearest convenience store. Grab some fruit or veggies; grab whatever is safest for you to nosh on and then get back to your dinner. I've left conference rooms during lunch breaks, I've run out to bodegas during birthday parties, and I've smiled my way through uneaten fish dinners in Barcelona. Never eat because you feel obligated.

The Salvageable Situation

Sometimes a restaurant experience can be brought back from the brink. The only way is to talk directly to the person who made the food: the chef. Here's an example. Due to scheduling conflicts, I missed my friend Allison's bachelorette party and shower, so I invited her to a special dinner, just the two of us. I took her to a spot I had been to a few times before with very safe results. I used an online reservation system and listed my allergies, and

I identified myself when I entered the restaurant. I was personally escorted to the table by the general manager, Oscar.

Once we were both seated, the restaurant assured me that they were aware of my requests and prepared to serve me a safe meal. However, our server let is slip that the chef was "worried" about my food-allergy needs. A worried chef equals a worried food-allergic diner. The server was doing his best to be responsible, but by the main course it became clear that the lines of communication had broken down. For instance, I was told that the cabbage had tree nuts in it and that my dish would be made without cabbage; however, my roasted hen showed up with a layer of cabbage underneath. Oscar came by to check on our table.

"I'm confused," I said. "I was told the cabbage wasn't safe for me."

"It's fine. I'm a thousand percent sure," he said.

"But I was told the cabbage was made with tree nuts. I'm scared to eat this."

Oscar said, "Come. Let's go see the chef." He took my hand, and we walked into the spotless kitchen. I met Chef Robert, who was expediting orders. He smiled broadly and reassured me that he was aware of all of my allergies and the cabbage only had caraway seeds; my meal was safe. I breathed a sigh of relief and returned to the table to eat.

Talking with the executive chef salvaged what had quickly become a confusing situation. The manager did exactly what he should have done: reassured me by taking me straight to the top. After cutting through the miscommunication, after meeting the chef, and after seeing the spotless kitchen, I had enough trust to be able to dine. The evening was saved.

That trust was solidified the next day when Oscar e-mailed me with his contact information, "Please e-mail me directly the next time you're planning to come in so I can take all of your fears away before you enter the restaurant."

Miscommunication with restaurant staff happens, and mistakes will happen. How you deal with them, how you restore trust in the dining experience, and how a restaurant handles the exchange are all factors in being able to dine successfully.

people with food allergies are the new VIPs

There's a trend that I've noticed: I call it "Allergies are the new VIP." Here is a recent example. I didn't know anyone in this restaurant, it was my first time dining there, and I didn't flash wads of cash. I just used the primer concepts in conjunction with the preparatory steps.

I was ushered into a New York institution's elegant front room, which was instantly familiar to me from two classic 1950s movies that were filmed there. I arrived early. Even though I had called ahead and told the manager about my allergies, I wanted to talk with the manager in person, out of earshot of my dining companions, since this was a work meeting. While waiting in the cocktail lounge, I saw my name and my allergies clearly spelled out in the reservation book. Excellent sign. I had a brief confirmation with the smiling manager, who assured me that the staff was ready for me (evidenced by the notes in his book).

When my party arrived, we were brought to our table, named "Bogie's Corner." Yes, Humphrey Bogart—and yes, his corner table, where he reportedly proposed to Lauren Bacall. Our knowledgeable server also had my allergies written down and memorized. He said the chef was prepared for me and would be happy to make any necessary accommodations to any dish I wanted. I ordered their famous burger made with duck fat. My bunless burger was fatty and rare, well seasoned, and yummy, and it arrived with complimentary steamed veggies, without my even having to ask. The general manger stopped by to check on our table several times; the server was solicitous and charming.

But then there was more. We were all laughing and drinking and eating when our excellent server came and asked me the best question of the night.

"Do you want to go downstairs?"

"Oh yes," I replied, without hesitation.

"What's downstairs?" my dinner companions asked. The secret wine cellar, of course, and we were in for a personal tour. We had a few minutes to wait while a group was finishing dining in there, so our server poured me a second glass of champagne, also complimentary, and we ate dessert (fresh berries for me). We toured the downstairs secret bootleg cellar, walking through the kitchen to get there. On the wall of the kitchen, I spied a list of the top eight most common allergens and what to do in case of an emergency. It felt like every step of the way, the red carpet was rolling out for our little group.

I left the restaurant wondering if this is how they treat everyone with allergies. I felt welcomed, I ate well, our server was a star, and there were no allergy issues. How did it all happen? I used the primer concepts and did all of the preparatory steps I've told you about.

worry-free dinners

All this happy dining out I do—five dinners a week and sometimes lunches and breakfasts, too—means that I use the primer concepts, the steps and these dining out strategies constantly. After years of using them and teaching them to private clients and blog readers, I decided that I wanted to share them on a larger scale, so I created Worry-Free Dinners.

Food-allergy awareness, clear communication, and communication practice create the kind of healthy two-way relationship required for restaurants and food-allergic patrons to engage one another positively. I launched Worry-Free Dinners, an arm of my private coaching practice, in February 2008 to help food-allergic families and food-allergic adults who have manageable food allergies to learn how to dine out safely and successfully.

The mission of Worry-Free Dinners is to teach members how to advocate for their dietary needs in different situations; to practice clear and effective communication skills; and to enjoy an allergen-friendly meal in the company of like-minded individuals. Worry-Free Dinners has members all over the country and restaurant group partnerships at multiple price points in multiple locations. Ultimately, Worry-Free Dinners is just one more option for the food-allergic community, a way to mix fun and education in a controlled restaurant setting. And there's always an allergy-free dessert on a Worry-Free Dinners menu.

An adult Worry-Free Dinners celiac member told me, "I thought it was really great to be able to sit down with a group of people [who] totally understand how I feel. I often feel alone in my anxiety about eating out and enjoying food, and it was so great to have that relieved for an evening."

This statement is from the mother of two children, seven and nine, who have multiple food allergies:

> Worry-Free Dinners gave my child a chance to eat restaurant food for the first time in his life. At bedtime, he declared that "eating at the restaurant was my favorite thing this weekend!" After spending time with other families and with Sloane, I have confidence that I could actually work with a restaurant staff to have a safe family meal out. We owe it all to Sloane for helping us take the leap, asking all the right questions and generally having the courage to do it.

Here's another quote from the mother of a fourteen-year-old girl, a multiple food-allergic child who had also never dined out in a restaurant before joining Worry-Free Dinners:

> We went to 7-Eleven for a Slurpee. Sounds pretty boring, but before the Worry-Free Dinners event, we wouldn't have done this. We asked the manager if

the Slurpee was free of milk, and he allowed us in the back of the store, where the ingredients are listed, to read it for ourselves. He was a very nice gentleman. We trusted and verified!

Dining out—whether with family, friends, on a date, or for work—is one of life's pleasures. When one has a dietary restriction, it can feel like a real burden. But you can carve out a space in between that is safe and fun. By engaging with a restaurant, by gathering information about who owns it and runs it and how these people want to interact with their patrons, you can find a restaurant that will serve you safely and well, that will work with you, that will embrace your food allergies, and where you will feel like a VIP, a food-allergic rock star. The first step is yours.

allergic girl's tips to reading the restaurant

- At every step of interacting with a restaurant you will acquire vital information. Listen, pay attention, and make an informed choice.
- Use the strategies described in this chapter. If you don't have time to do them in advance, do them on-site.
- Communicate your needs early and often, and be your most charming self. If that isn't mirrored by a restaurant's staff, take your business elsewhere.
- Restaurants are in the hospitality business; they should be doing their best to welcome you. If they aren't doing their job, take your business elsewhere.
- If you can't leave, for some reason, do your best to find an ally at your table or within the restaurant.
- Remember the backup plans: keep safe snacks on you, nosh ahead of the dinner, and have your medication on you at all times.

- Nationally, more and more restaurants and restaurant chains are catering to the food-allergic diner. Take advantage of these programs by patronizing these restaurants. If they do a good job, give them feedback. If they don't, let them know that, too.
- The Worry-Free Dinners program is a resource for the food-allergy community. Together we practice all of the strategies outlined in this book. Visit Allergicgirl.com for more information about Worry-free Dinners.

12

unstoppable

It's when you're safe at home that you wish you
were having an adventure. When you're having an
adventure, you wish you were safe at home.
—Thornton Wilder

Balmy breezes, white-sandy beaches, and swaying palms; I
can taste the rum punch already. Or tall glass towers and
bustling streets below, with millions of stories around every corner; I can't wait to eavesdrop. I love the adventure of being somewhere new and getting to know the local people, the traditions,
the sights, the surroundings, the history, and the culture.

Even better, I like creating my regular routine somewhere new.
Quotidian details can transform a mere visit into a lasting stay:
drinking Prosecco wine from a tap like a Venetian; talking with
the Amish cheese purveyor in Philadelphia's Redding Market
about his prized cows; getting a *carnet* in Paris and riding the

rails—feeling like a regular and not just a tourist. That's my favorite part of traveling.

My least favorite part of traveling is the travel. I'm more of a *stayer* than a traveler. I'm a really good stayer.

travel concerns

Everyone loves to travel. I can fall under its shiny lure, too. When I'm home, I dream of going away, but when I'm sitting on the tarmac, I wonder, "Whose bright idea was this?"

What I don't love about travel is the getting there, especially when it intersects with my food allergies, which is all the time. The prospect of having a food-allergy reaction thirty-five thousand feet in the air doesn't thrill me. There are nuts everywhere, the air is recycled, the seats aren't cleaned, and people bring scary foods from home and snack during the flight (walnut cream cheese on a bagel, anyone?). If I become allergic during a flight, where do I go for relief? What if the medications don't help? Or worse, what if I forgot to put my medications in my carry-on bag? Will the pilot land the plane for me? (How mortifying!)

That's a planeload of claustrophobia in a tin can right there. And that's just the start. When I get to where I'm going, what am I going to eat? How am I going to get something safe? How often will I be able to get it? What if the people don't speak English, and my Franglish, Spanglish, Italianish, or Chinesish is too laughable to be understood? It's hard enough in my own country; now do I have to be an international food-allergic person?

When I'm traveling for business, what if I'm making my presentation and the conference center has only vending machines with nutty candies, and other noncomestibles? What if the business dinner with the boss is at the local Thai restaurant, with nothing to eat but fish in fish sauce—now what? Do I just drink water? To whom could I talk discreetly, without making a scene? What if, what if, what if? It can all spiral into no-fun land.

For Healthcentral.com, I interviewed Robert Haru Fisher, an editor of Frommers.com and a professional travel writer. He's anaphylactically allergic to peanuts and some legumes. He told me the following story:

> Once on a domestic flight, I had preordered the peanut-free meal. However, the moment I took my first bite, I realized something was wrong: it had peanuts in it. I immediately drank some liquid Benadryl and injected my thigh with the Epi-Pen. I informed the airline stewardess of the situation and, luckily, didn't feel the need to ask [the crew] to land the plane. We landed, and I went home, self-medicated, and rested, and it went away. These severe reactions to peanuts didn't happen until I was already an adult in my thirties. I already knew what I wanted to do in my life, which was travel and write. I wasn't going to let anything stop me, not even a life-threatening allergy. I love what I do; I love seeing what's around the next corner.

Robert has true wanderlust; he loves what he does and is not going to let anything stop him. His attitude is one that anybody with severe food allergies could borrow when traveling: not being stopped by food allergies.

basic needs when traveling

Being in and of the world is the ultimate goal for those of us with dietary restrictions. Traveling is about being literally in and of the world, about leaving your safe zone and getting out there. For anyone with a chronic medical condition, traveling away from the safe zone quickly becomes an issue of getting one's basic needs met in multiple situations and scenarios, some known and some unknown, in order to have the best time possible.

For me, the basic needs are getting to a destination food allergy–free and remaining food allergen–free while staying there, eating both well and safely. When those needs are met, I can enjoy the destination, see the attractions, and get a feel for the local flavor. I make that happen by instituting specific homework, planning ahead, making smart choices on-site, and using the primer concepts and strategies we've discussed all along the way. Think briefly about your most basic needs when you're traveling, and keep them in mind as we move through this section.

planning a trip

Planning a trip, for some people, is the best part of a vacation; for some it's the part they dread, avoid, or farm out. A *New York Times* article on February 18, 2010, cited a Dutch study that found that many people were happiest when planning a trip (they were less happy about actually being on the trip).

Tap into the happy excitement about planning. Envision yourself having a grand old time; think of good weather, easy flights, welcoming hotels, and restaurants that embrace food allergies. Get excited about your trip and allow the unknowns to equal possibility, not disappointment. If you're not a planner, become one. If you really don't have a talent for organization, train yourself to be organized about this one thing—your health can depend on it. If you really hate planning and organizing, hire someone or ask a friend who loves to plan and offer something in exchange.

be spontaneous

I'm all for spontaneity; however, anyone with a condition that could become life-threatening must take the most basic precautions:

- Always have your medications on hand and make sure they are up to date.
- Bring trusted over-the-counter medications with you.

- Download mobile phone applications that have your allergies described in other languages.
- Carry a laminated card in your wallet with instructions on what to do in an emergency.
- Wear a medical alert bracelet with your allergies described.
- Program ICE (in case of emergency) numbers into your cell phone. Examples: ICE mom, ICE sister, ICE spouse, ICE allergist.

Whether at home or away, *you are your best first responder*.

pre-trip homework

If you want to do some pre-trip homework (or are a type A planner), then go wild with the suggestions here. You needn't to do all of them to have a successful and safe trip, but you should do some of them. Pick and choose, depending on the situation. The difference in the outcome of your trip, in terms of safety and fun, will be immeasurable. Some are more time- and labor-intensive, and some can be accomplished with a phone call or just a few clicks of your mouse. Above all, have realistic expectations for what will happen while you are away. Being away from home is not like being at home, and it shouldn't be. Enjoy the foreign nature of it and the adventure, but don't expect it to be like home.

Here's a story of how just a little bit of homework before a cruise paid off for a Worry-Free Dinners member with celiac disease and food allergies:

> For my birthday vacation, my parents and I went on a cruise to Alaska. My mom chose a cruise company that has a food needs form for booked guests. I filled out the form and spoke with the booking agent about my dietary needs. The agent told me that I would be able to keep my own homemade yogurt in the refrigerator behind the bar. They even have a gluten-free option on

the initial form. When I arrived on the ship, the second mate found me and brought the chef up to meet with me. He was absolutely great. He had read all my notes and fully understood my limitations. Every morning after breakfast, the chef found me and we discussed the day's menu, what I wanted to have, and how he could prepare it. For my birthday, rather than making a cake for my table to share, he made a great fruit purée with no sugar or dairy for me and everyone at my table. It was so wonderful to be so well taken care of and not to have to worry about what kind of food I was going to get. I didn't need to eat any of my emergency food until we left the ship. I know there were other diners with restrictions and allergies who got the same kind of attention as well.

It's not a lot of work—not any more than typing your needs onto a form and following up on-site. And saying thank you—easily done, and the results far outweigh the work involved.

The Internet

Start where most homework begins these days: the Internet. Whether you're Googling from your cell phone, using Bing from your laptop, or accessing the free computers at the library, look up your destination. Type the name of the city into the search engine of choice, and the city's chamber of commerce or the city's government site will pop up. This is great place to start, as a portal to other reputable and reliable sites. Find out the local weather, what's fun to do, the local drinking and eating spots, and historical sites and attractions. Most important, look up the contact information for local hospitals, allergy centers, and medical or nursing centers.

Local Food-Allergy Groups

Use the Internet to search for food-allergy support groups and meetings in your destination city. These support groups have a wealth of information about the area and are highly motivated to help people with food allergies who are coming to town. Browse the site; it may have local restaurant and doctor listings or a FAQ section that will answer your questions. If you don't find what you're looking for, then e-mail the group leader directly.

Here's a sample e-mail for a local allergy group:

> Dear Food Allergy Group of Atlanta,
>
> I'm planning on visiting Atlanta this summer. I'm so excited! However, I'm allergic to salmon and all tree nuts, and I'm wondering if you or your members know of any great local restaurants or hotels that cater to those of us with dietary restrictions. Any assistance would be greatly appreciated. I can be reached by e-mail or cell phone [contact info provided]. Thank you in advance!
>
> Best wishes,
>
> Sloane Miller

Do this well in advance of your trip in order to give someone ample time to respond.

Your Library or Bookstore

Use your library or bookstore to find travel books or magazines about your destination; read them and get to know the place. Talk to the librarians; they typically have tons of great information and know the library inside and out. Look up books about the cuisine of your destination. Whether you're looking for Tex-Mex or Laotian, there's a cookbook about every popular ethnic and regional cuisine. Familiarize yourself with the names of traditional dishes that could be problematic so you can identify them when you see them on a menu.

AAA

The American Automobile Association (AAA) isn't just for your grandparents. AAA's TripTik and map system is an excellent and underutilized resource if you are driving to your destination. AAA has listings of local attractions and hospitals all in a handy and free guide that is included in AAA membership, which is a bargain if you travel by car frequently. It also offers travel insurance, something to think about that we will discuss more later.

Local Tourism Boards

Whether you're going abroad or staying stateside, tourism boards exist for many of the most popular travel destinations. Call or e-mail to get their free brochures. You can also call them and ask about local restaurants and attractions. These people are paid to talk about your destination. Use them and their knowledge.

Consulates

Are you going outside the United States, including Mexico or Canada? If you live in or near a big city, you can march right in to the consulate of your destination country without an appointment and talk to someone about your trip. If you don't live near a consulate, call one and ask about your destination. People who work in consulates usually love to talk about their home countries, so give them a chance to brag and help you out at the same time.

Ethnic Restaurants

Ethnic restaurants in your hometown can be a resource to prepare you for going abroad. If you're going to Thailand, Mexico, China, or Japan, for example, visit a Thai, Mexican, Chinese, or Japanese restaurant in your hometown and talk with the owners, the managers, or the staff. They'll tell you what you can eat when you visit their home countries and what to avoid.

Be considerate of their time, however: it's best to do this during off-hours, such as midafternoon or late at night, when the staff won't be extremely busy with customers and can take the time to chat with you.

Local Medical Professionals and Hospitals

Ask your doctor or allergist for a medical referral in the area to which you're traveling. It's nice to have the name of a local doctor who's well liked among his or her peers. Five-star hotels and local U.S. consulates are another source of finding American or English-speaking doctors in a foreign country, once you're there, but it's best to have this information ahead of time. Have the names and addresses of the local hospitals and emergency rooms handy. If you are going to need a prescription filled while you're away, remember that your home doctor can't call that in for you once you leave home.

Health Insurance

There are several ways to guarantee that you have basic coverage while you're traveling, depending on your budget and your needs. Your credit card company, your managed-care provider, Medic Alert, and AAA all offer coverage and are good places to start. Sometimes an alumni association, a professional association, and even your place of employment will have special travel coverage. If you have homeowner's or renter's insurance, that might cover travel, too.

business travel

When you're traveling for business, you may feel a lack of control over where and when they send you. However, you can still apply many of the planning suggestions above as soon as you know where you are going. Contact your company's travel agency and start helping them to help you.

Be Gutsy

Take control of the part of the traveling situation that you have access to so that you can get your food-allergy needs met. Once those needs are met, you'll be able to concentrate fully on the task at hand. Connect to your food-allergy needs without shame, embarrassment, and apology; communicate those needs clearly, assertively, and graciously; and recognize that you have options and that there is always a way to get what you need.

If you think that you don't have the guts to do this yet in a work scenario, borrow mine—I have plenty. Seriously; think "What would Allergic Girl do?" when you're attempting to do this for the first time. Or think of your favorite gutsy characters in a movie, a play, or a book or on TV. What would they do or say to get what they need in a way that you respect and think you could emulate? Become them just for a moment. Borrow one of their personas and try it on for size. You might find that you like it, and you might find that it helps you to get what you need.

Call Ahead

Find out who's doing the corporate trip planning and reach out. Call first and follow up with an e-mail to confirm how you've both decided to proceed. Starting with a call is the best way to get a positive reply, such as "Yes, we can handle that right away." E-mails can get buried and may be perceived as more work for the recipient.

Here's a sample phone conversation with multiple options. Keep it light, friendly, and nonaggressive. Remember, you're looking for the person's help.

> Good morning, Sally, I'm Sloane. I am scheduled for a trip
> to San Diego for a conference from April sixteenth to

the nineteenth. I have severe food allergies, so I need to do some planning before I head off, and I'm hoping you can help me. How does your department normally handle these requests? I don't want to make more work for you, so I'm happy to do all of the special arrangements myself. I'd be happy to make some calls to the airlines or the hotels. Can you tell me where we're booked? Alternatively, I can send you my list of needs. Sometimes it's easier for me to deal directly with the hotel or the conference center or the caterer, but I'm happy to send you a detailed list of my needs, if your department works best that way. When and how should I follow up? With whom should I follow up? I will follow up with them or you or your manager by e-mail. Thank you!

Here's a sample post-phone call follow-up e-mail:

Dear Sally,

Great chatting with you just now. I really appreciate your help. It will allow me to fully concentrate on my work once I know these details are taken care of. Here's a rundown of what we just discussed: I'm scheduled to travel with the editorial department to San Diego for a sales conference from April sixteenth to the nineteenth. I have some medical needs: I'm allergic to tree nuts, fish, and shellfish and need some assistance planning meals ahead of time. We discussed that you would call the conference center and I would deal with the hotel and the restaurant where we have our big sales dinner. I will follow up with you by phone in two weeks. Until then, I'm here to help!

Thank you in advance,

Sloane

Offer to Help

Reread the previous section. Offer to do as much as you can yourself, like calling the airline for a special meal or calling the conference center. If there is a special dinner planned, get the name of the manager and call him or her directly to convey your needs, so you're not stuck with your boss and the seafood-allergic person's nightmare, the pupu platter.

packing

If you pack just one thing, make it your up-to-date, emergency medications in your purse, carry-on bag, briefcase, school bag, or messenger bag. Here are some additional packing tips for bringing a little "home sweet (and safe) home" with you wherever you go.

Check your medications. Did I mention it's important to bring your medication? I'm talking about both your prescriptions and your favorite over-the-counter meds. Before you leave, take the time to go through your travel medicine kit. Is everything up-to-date? Do you need doubles or triples of anything? Do you have enough medication if an inhaler is left in a hotel or a pill case is dropped in the lavatory? Talk with your doctor about what medications he or she recommends that you have in your travel kit. Do not take shortcuts with this step.

Bring snacks. We call them travel snacks, in my family. On a long car ride, plane ride, or train ride, safe travel snacks are necessary. If you are traveling in a car or on a train, you can bring a cooler, but otherwise nonperishable snacks are a must. On my first transatlantic flight, when I was eleven, we brought a picnic basket. Do what you need to do here to ensure that you have safe food while you're in transit.

Send food ahead. If you're traveling somewhere and you think you won't be able to find anything to eat there, or they don't have a great supermarket or a farmer's market, or you're simply feeling unsure, send some food ahead. FedEx, UPS, and the postal service will ship nonperishables or perishables anywhere in the world. You can ask the hotel where you're staying to hold on to the package for you, if you let the staff know ahead of time that goodies are arriving. Buy your food directly from a special online food retailer and have it sent where you're going. Is there a Whole Foods where you're visiting? It might deliver to your destination; call and find out. If you need a lot of food where you're traveling, send the food ahead. Just get it there.

Take chef cards. When you're dining on the road, away from home, laminated allergy chef cards are a great help. They outline your allergies, using words and pictures, and you can even get them in other languages, which is great for traveling abroad or eating in ethnic restaurants. A few companies have created cell phone applications that essentially do the same thing, so there's no excuse for not having chef cards in your wallet or on your phone. Do an Internet search for ones that suit your phone and carrier.

Bring medical alert jewelry. When I went overseas for a year during college, I got my first medical alert bracelet, and I've had it ever since. There are several companies on the market now that make them in all price ranges and for all ages. Talk with your medical Team You about whether it's appropriate for you to get one and also which one is preferable.

getting there

Now that you've done your trip-planning homework, let's talk about the getting-there part.

Cars

The road trip is as American as any of our most treasured institutions, like democracy, baseball, and apple pie (tree nut-free, of course). For the food-allergic community, this American pastime is the easiest solution when traveling: a road trip gives you the most control. Where you go, how much money you spend, your route, and where and how often you stop along the way are all choices that are entirely up to you. Food is less of an issue because you can take it with you. For the food-allergic community, car travel is the golden standard for traveling in the Unites States and abroad.

An Emergency Kit for the Car

If you have decided to get your kicks while driving on Route 66, don't overlook basic car care before you travel: check the oil, tire pressure, brake fluid, battery gauge, lights, and gas tank. Not a car person? Ask your mechanic or your car dealership to give your car the once-over before any long trip.

Take along the following items:

- Car battery chargers that charge themselves.
- Standard safety kits for traveling; these are available online, at major outlets, at supersaver stores, and at large sales clubs. Get one and customize it with food-allergy medications, drinks, and snacks.
- Chargers for your laptop, cell phones, music devices, and plug-in, portable coolers.
- Allergy-friendly pillows and blankets; these are great for car travel and transition easily if your hotel doesn't haven't any safe blankets and pillows.
- Shelf-stable ultra-high-temperature (UHT) products: milk or dairy-free milk alternatives, safe granola bars, cheese and cracker packs; keep them in the trunk.
- Music, DVDs, word puzzles, books you've been meaning to read (or audio books you've been meaning to listen to).
- Your sense of adventure.

A Global Positioning System

Many newer-model cars off the lot come with a global positioning system (GPS) built in. However, for anywhere between fifty and two hundred dollars, you can buy a portable unit to use when you travel in a rental car or another vehicle. GPS devices have local hospitals and health care centers, as well as chain restaurants, programmed in; I love that feature. So if you have a chain restaurant that you know is safe for you, you can find an outpost along your route for safe meals. Many cell phones now have incredibly useful GPS systems or map applications.

Meds and Cars

I leave an autoinjector, an inhaler, and some antihistamines in the glove compartment of my car and check them every month or so. When I check them, I take them out, inspect them for damage, check the date, see that the pills haven't melted, and look at the color of the liquid in the autoinjector. If the liquid is not clear, throw the autoinjector away and replace it immediately.

If you're traveling or living somewhere exceedingly hot or cold, then don't leave your meds in the car, because heat and cold can adversely affect medications, especially epinephrine, the contents of autoinjectors. Keep them in a travel kit that you take to and from the car.

Lifesaving medicine must be with you *at all times.* Evan Edwards one of the developers of the Intelliject epinephrine autoinjector, had a very close call. He didn't have an epinephrine autoinjector with him when he had a reaction at a restaurant. It was in his car. Fortunately, the local hospital was just minutes away. Do not let this happen to you; you might not be as fortunate.

Trains

For most long-distance, interstate train travel in the United States, you'll be boarding an Amtrak train. Amtrak has joined this century by having a lot of online information, including how it accommodates special diets like kosher, vegetarian, and vegan in its dining cars. It doesn't have allergen-friendly or gluten-free menus (yet), but call ahead of time and see what it can offer. If you have any lingering concerns, bring your trusty cooler and your own safe meals.

Planes

We're in the middle of a paradigm shift regarding airline travel and food allergies. As more and more Americans are diagnosed with life-threatening food allergies, the airlines are working hard on policies about how to handle the overwhelming requests for peanut-free flights (no one's tackled tree nuts yet). However, it's undeniable that airline policy on airborne food allergens seems to change weekly. Different airlines in different hubs in different countries handle these issues and customer requests differently. As of this writing, there is no one unifying policy or statement that anyone can make about how to handle airline travel for people with food allergies, mainly because no carrier can control what other passengers do, nor will any carrier ever guarantee your safety.

Do your best to ensure your own safety. Talk with your medical Team You about what is right for you and how to keep yourself safe when traveling by air. Do some pre-trip homework about your carrier and assess the best course of action for you.

The Good and the Not-So-Good of Airline Travel

We all have stories (or have heard them or read them) about how different airlines handle food-allergy requests. Allergic Girl colleague Elizabeth Landau of CNN.com (who is allergic to tree nuts, peanuts, artichokes, and seafood) told me the following about flying. Like many of us, she has experienced airlines that handled her needs well and airlines that have lost her trust and business.

Some people get jittery on planes because they fear a crash landing. I, on the other hand, have sat on the edge of my seat dozens of times worrying about people around me chewing peanuts and getting dust in the air that could make my mouth itch or, even worse, [make me] go into anaphylaxis. I fly frequently to see friends and family members around the country, so this has always been a real issue. On several trips, even after I explained my allergy, flight attendants have refused to stop serving peanuts, insisting that they are obligated to give out these snacks. I remember one time my mom had to spell out that it's easier to stop serving peanuts than to take the plane down in a medical emergency, and only then did the flight attendant take away packets of peanuts she'd already given out around me. We called the airline afterward to complain and received a voucher toward our next flight, as a consolation. But we booked our return flight on a different carrier, as I no longer trusted it. I didn't fly with that airline again until it changed its policy to preclude serving peanuts. There seems to be some movement toward understanding on an official level at various airlines, but it doesn't always work in practice. On a recent flight, even though I notified three different people involved in my travel process, the flight attendant in charge of my section failed to recognize the peanut-free zone I had been promised.

Finding which airline will refrain from serving nutty snacks to anyone at all, if this is necessary for your safety, is an arduous process. *Allergic Living* magazine (www.allergicliving.com/documents/airlines.asp) created a foldout of eight major airline carriers and their allergen policies. It'll give you a good start. Policies change, so before you make any flight reservations, check with the carrier directly.

Airborne Allergens

One of the main concerns of many food allergic people is that when traveling by plane, they may be confronted by their allergen, also along for the ride. I asked Dr. Matthew Greenhawt to explain some of the basic airborne allergy issues:

> Despite reports from allergic individuals that aerosolized peanut dust can trigger a reaction, three studies show otherwise. The first study aimed to determine if peanut allergen could be found circulating in the cabin air of an airplane, and [it] did find detectible levels of the major peanut allergen in the air filter. This study did not examine the effects of this on passengers. A second study investigated the effect of topical and inhalational exposure to a surface containing peanut butter to peanut-allergic children. No symptoms were reported from these exposures.
>
> Because peanut butter is less likely to aerosolize than peanut dust or flour, the final study investigated different environmental routes of peanut exposure. These included opening bags of unshelled peanuts or roasted shelled peanuts, opening peanut butter, and stepping on peanut shells on a floor within an enclosed space with both good and poor ventilation (simulating airborne exposure at a sporting event and in an approximated airplane cabin). No peanut allergen was detected in the air samples. As a result of this data, many reported inhalational exposures have been viewed with skepticism. Many investigators attribute inhalational exposure to unintentional ingestion of trace peanut dust or residue. Though every peanut-allergic individual should take the appropriate precautions to limit their exposure through contact or inhalation in public settings, the data shows that there is a limited risk of reaction due to encounters via these routes of exposure.

If you must fly and you have concerns, have a frank discussion with your medical Team You about the real risks for you.

being there

Once you've done the traveling part, now comes the fun part: actually staying there. The hospitality industry has many names for your temporary accomodations: hotel, motel, inn, *pensione*, *auberge*, spa, resort, or bed-and-breakfast. Any lodging away from home will be your new "home" for a few days and you'll be in the capable hands of members of the hospitality industry. Here's the most important point to remember about the hospitality industry: its their job is to make you feel welcomed. Give its employees the chance to do that by letting them know what you need in advance. This is where all of the excellent homework you've done will come into play.

Hotels, Motels, and More

I asked hotelier Matthew V. Moore, director of rooms and environmental programs at the Seaport Hotel and Seaport World Trade Center in Boston, what's reasonable to ask for, in terms of accommodations for an allergic traveler, from the hotel's perspective.

"I think there are a few accommodations that can be made for those traveling with allergies," he said, "like calling ahead and inquiring if the culinary team at the hotel's restaurants has specialized menus for those with food allergies. At the very least, ask if the hotel has a staff that is knowledgeable and creative enough to provide options to those who would need them. It's important that the guest doesn't have to compromise on luxury or comfort just because of their allergies."

Keep that in mind when choosing a hotel and when checking in. You have the right, just like anyone else, to comfort and even luxury when traveling and staying away from home.

kitchen with a side of hotel

Most national hotel chains (Hyatt, Loews, Marriott, Double-tree, Embassy Suites, Holiday Inn) have either extended-stay hotels or suites with kitchen facilities. You should be able to find a suite within your budget in most major U.S. cities. Having a kitchenette or a full kitchen is a boon for the food-allergic traveler. Even if you can't find a suite or a hotel room with a kitchen, many hotels will bring up an extra empty fridge on request (usually with no charge).

Before Check-In

Whether you're staying in a large hotel chain or a small bed-and-breakfast, there's a human to deal with in there somewhere. Sometimes you will have to press a few buttons on the telephone to get to someone, but it's worth it. Get to that human, tell him or her your food-allergy needs, and write down the person's name and when the two of you spoke. Ask for an e-mail confirmation of your requests.

If you can't find a human to deal with, there's often a section for notes when you're booking online. Put your food-allergy requests there, and follow up when you check in. You can also ask for the concierge.

The Concierge

Concierges have specialized training within the hospitality indus-try to know more about their local areas and attractions as well as the inner working of the hotel in which they work. The inter-national concierge membership organization is Les Clefs d'Or, or the Golden Keys; look for the crossed-key pin on their lapels to know you're dealing with top professionals in the field. Concierges are an underutilized resource when you have any special dietary requests or room requests. For example, if you haven't spoken with your hotel's chef yet or feel shy about calling him or her directly, your hotel's concierge can facilitate that exchange. This person can also to put you in touch with the hotel's director of rooms, the general manager, or housekeeping to help make your stay as allergen friendly as possible. This is a free service provided by the hotel; use it to your advantage.

If you just want some help getting to know your local destination better and your hotel does not have a concierge, go into any top-rated hotel (a five-star is preferable), and talk to the concierge. You don't have to be staying at the hotel to talk with its concierge. Use the new sunny attitude you've been practicing and find out all you need to know, especially about any local restaurant that may be good with food allergies.

Check-In

Try to check in early so you'll have your pick of the available rooms. When you arrive, gently remind the front-desk staff of any special requests. When you get into your room, if you find that your requests weren't honored, get a different room. If you don't like your room—it smells of smoke or cleaning fluid, it hasn't been cleaned properly, it's near the ice machine, or anything that doesn't seem right—switch. Don't settle; call the front desk and tell the staffperson that you're not happy with your room and you want another room. Remember, honey works better than vinegar, but make it a firm request.

Empty the Hotel Fridge

If you didn't book ahead or you couldn't find a hotel with kitchen facilities, then try to book a hotel room with a minibar. Once you're inside, empty out the minibar and fill it with your own allergy-friendly goodies. Tell the hotel before you do this so it doesn't charge you for all the hotel treats you didn't eat, and make sure to refill the minibar with everything before you leave.

Even better, before you arrive, request an empty fridge on arrival. Hotels will often accommodate that request.

Hotel Kitchen Staff

Make friends with the hotel's kitchen staff and chef; get them on your side by using the primer concepts. A quick friendly conversation with the chef of your hotel's kitchen and you may find an unexpected ally. Create that rapport, and your new chefy friend might even make you your favorite allergen-friendly meal. Be clear about your food-allergic needs, and again, be sure to use lots of pleases and thank-yous! (A monetary thanks when you leave is always appreciated, as well.)

Check Out the Hotel Guide

The hotel guide in your room will probably have names of local hospitals and local medical professionals. If you are feeling nervous about your destination, take some of that fear away by checking in with the hotel doctor or nurse. I don't know of one hotel that doesn't have a medical professional on staff or on call. Even if you are staying in a *pensione* or a youth hostel, these places have names of local medical professionals for travelers.

If you find it necessary, give the medical professional a call, find out his or her fees and hours, and explain your needs. Just check in. It's better to do it routinely than in an emergency. Knowing a local medical professional can come in handy, especially if you need a prescription filled locally. Remember, your hometown general practitioner or allergist can't call in an out-of-state prescription. If you need a monthly prescription or your prescription was lost or stolen, it's good to have a doctor on hand locally.

Give Feedback

If the hotel does a great job with your room and your special dietary requests, fill out the response form in the room or follow up after you leave with a kind letter to management (e-mail is fine). Tell the hotel management who, specifically, helped you and how. Hotels need your feedback. For the hotel staff members who helped you, your compliment or thank-you goes into their permanent records.

Conversely, if everyone was just plain mean, incompetent, confused, or absent, then tell the hotel that, too. Speak up before you leave. Let the manager know specifically what went wrong: the room was dirty, the food was awful or unsafe, and the staff incompetent. The hotel should try to make it up to you monetarily, by taking the tax off the bill or offering a free night or free parking. When you stay at a hotel, you're paying for a service. If the service is poor, you shouldn't be paying a premium for it. Also, the hotel wants you back. It is in the hospitality industry, and it works best, here or around the world, when you are a repeat customer.

Think of any hotel chain in the United States: Marriott, Holiday Inn, Hilton, Ritz-Carlton, Hyatt, Four Seasons. They are worldwide brands. If you have a good experience at one franchise, the odds are that you will want to book with the chain again elsewhere. Give a hotel the chance to treat you well. Communicate your needs, follow up, take names, and rebook.

dining out while traveling

All of the strategies covered in chapter 11 will work when you're traveling. However, here are some extra tips to consider when you're outside your comfort zone.

Shop Locally

Go food shopping at the local green market or farmers' market. This is a great way to get to know the area and pick up seasonal and fresh produce. Find local health-food stores or supermarket chains that stock allergen-friendly foods you can eat. Get to know local shop merchants, local foods, and local specialties. You can often learn more about a culture through what it eats than the art it hangs on the walls. Whether you're in New London, Connecticut, or London, England, there will be something to be learned by food shopping. Go for it: get local.

Dine In

As I mentioned previously, your hotel chef can be one of the best hidden resources for dining with food allergies away from home. Hotel chefs are usually highly trained and deal with special food requests daily; it's another great resource right at your virtual door when staying away from home. For example, talking with the hotel chef is usually the second thing I do after checking into my room. Because of my food allergies, I have made hotel chef contacts all over the world who go out of their way to make me feel welcome and safe by creating special "Sloane meals." I make that happen by using the primer concepts and the dining out strategies in chapter 11. For some extra tips, I spoke with Chef Cliff Saladin of the Sheraton Tarrytown Hotel in New York about his guidelines for guests who wish to dine in his hotel, and he told me the following:

- When making a reservation for your hotel room, in the section for "notes," tell the staff what you need and ask them to make the kitchen aware of your food allergies or food restrictions.
- When you arrive at the hotel, make yourself known to the hotel chef.
- When you're dining in the hotel, give them at least twenty-four hours' notice of your needs.
- Please, bring a chef card detailing your allergies. It takes the mystery out of it and eliminates surprises.
- Above all: We are here for you, the guest, so let us know what you need.

Chef Cliff said that what helped him the most was my telling him exactly what I wanted for lunch and for dinner. You might think that some chefs wouldn't want to be told exactly what to make or how to make it. That's certainly true for some chefs, who want to give you what *they* determine you need. But more and more, the attitude is "We are here for you; tell us how to feed you." So go and tell them—nicely and graciously, but do it.

Use Translated Chef Cards

As we discussed in chapter 11, there are companies that will create chef cards or allergy cards that list your allergies and even include pictures to hand to a chef or server when dining out. Several of those card companies have them available in multiple languages for traveling. Get them and use them. Most of the executive chefs I've spoken to and interviewed, like Chef Cliff, have said that they like them because they are so clear, and they "eliminate the surprise."

However, as in all things, but especially when you are traveling away from your safe zone, even if you've done all of the steps and and if you still don't trust your meal, don't eat it. I am giving you permission right now. There is no shame in listening to your intuition and finding that it says, "I don't trust this meal."

Once you get comfortable utilizing the concepts strategies in this book, and finding your own spin on them, you'll find that you'll be better able to trust both your intuition and those who are serving you a safe meal.

be unstoppable

Some of my most memorable life experiences have been traveling and eating well. When I was eight, a sailboat captain showed me all of the stages of the coconut fruit in St. Maarten (coconut jelly, coconut water—yum). There was a T-shirt my mom bought for me in Paris when I was eleven that had Mickey Mouse saying, "Je suis allergique," with a picture of the Eiffel Tower in the background. When I was fifteen, in Venice, Italy, the *pensione* owner made me a special vegetarian *allergico* plate of fresh local cheese and fruit. I can still remember the vegan lentil salad that the kosher butcher's wife made for me in Juan-Les-Pins, France, when I was twenty.

Just last year, on a business trip for Worry-Free Dinners, the restaurant's general manager in Stowe, Vermont, had severe peanut allergies, and he took care of my meals personally. Even more recently, at the Natural Products Expo East conference, I met two women at the hotel bar, both of whom, coincidentally, had food allergies—we had a long giggle about the coincidences of that.

I had all of these life experiences because I connect to my food-allergy needs without shame, embarrassment, and apology; I communicate those needs clearly, assertively, and graciously; and I recognize that I have options and that there is always a way to get what I need. You too now have the confidence, the language, the attitude, and the tools to keep yourself safe in every situation.

Go, do, and see what's around the next corner. Be unstoppable.

allergic girl's launching pad

- Flexibility, a sense of humor, safe snacks, and your emergency medications are the barest minimum to bring along with you when traveling.
- It's vital to talk with your medical Team You about your food allergy risks and what precautions to take when traveling *before you go*.
- Traveling for vacation is supposed to be fun and enjoyable. By using the strategies in this book and doing some pre-trip homework, you can access the fun while managing your food allergy risk and staying safe.

- If you are traveling for work, find allies within the company and ensure that you are traveling as comfortably and as safely as possible.
- Remember, there's a fine line between trying to control everything (which is impossible) and taking reasonable care of your needs (which is entirely possible). It will take trial and error and time to create that balance; but keep chipping away at it.
- Ultimately, staying safe, taking care of yourself and your food allergy needs when you're traveling away from home is a great source of personal pride. Honor that part of yourself; he or she has done a great job.

epilogue

It's an early spring morning. New York City is just waking up. The sun is rising over the East River with a pink glow and the traffic on Second Avenue is still light. I've been writing at my desk an hour already, sipping Earl Grey tea and planning out the day ahead of me.

I still have to blog about last night's dinner. The chef made me a completely allergen-free dessert. I think I'm in love with him and his dessert. I have a lunch meeting with a Worry-Free Dinners event partner chef to try out her new menu ideas and items. The chef has a list of my allergies, but I'll remind her again and since I've switched purses today, I need to double-check that I have all of my meds.

Later, I'm cashing in a birthday present for spa services at my favorite salon, where my allergies are spelled out in the computer file and the spa products are tree nut free. Massage and mani-pedi without hives, how excellent. I need to e-mail Stéphanie about Passover at her house later this month: what can I bring, what is she serving, when do we eat?

Tonight I have a cocktail event for a restaurant opening with Shari and Francine; I hope the cute restaurateur is there. Then I'm dropping by a birthday celebration at a chic Asian fusion restaurant for Steve. I have leftovers from last night's allergen-free dinner to eat beforehand and some tree-nut-free homemade granola and organic dried apricots in my bag as backup. It's a fairly typical day, and food allergies are a consideration but only one among many because I'm confident that I can take care of my food allergy needs in any situation and have a great time while doing so.

My hope is that through this journey we've taken together and that with these new concepts, tips, and strategies, you now have the tools to be in and of the world with a little more trust, a little more faith, and a whole lot more fun.

resources

The Allergic Girl Web site contains up-to-the-minute information, more stories and strategies, reliable links to further resources, information about Worry-Free Dinners, and much more. Visit me at http://allergicgirl.com or e-mail me at sloane.miller @allergicgirl.com.

Allergic Living magazine
2100 Bloor Street West
Suite 6-168
Toronto, Ontario M6S 5A5
Canada
1 (888) 771-7747
www.allergicliving.com

American Academy of Allergy,
Asthma, and Immunology
555 East Wells Street
Suite 1100
Milwaukee, WI 53202-3823
(414) 272-6071
info@aaaai.org

American College of Allergy,
Asthma, and Immunology
85 West Algonquin Road

Suite 550
Arlington Heights, IL 60005
(847) 427-1200
mail@acaai.org
http://www.acaai.org/

American Dietetic Association
120 South Riverside Plaza
Suite 2000
Chicago, IL 60606-6995
1 (800) 877-1600
www.mypyramid.gov
www.eatright.org

American Medical Association
515 North State Street
Chicago, IL 60654
1 (800) 621-8335
www.ama-assn.org

American Psychological
 Association (APA)
750 First Street, NE
Washington, DC 20002-4242
(800) 374-2721
www.apa.org

American Psychiatric Association
 (APA)
1000 Wilson Boulevard
Suite 1825
Arlington, VA 22209
(888) 35-PSYCH
www.psych.org

Anaphylaxis Canada
2005 Sheppard Avenue East
Suite 800
Toronto, Ontario M2J 5B4
Canada
1 (866) 785-5660
www.anaphylaxis.ca

Asthma and Allergy Foundation
 of America
8201 Corporate Drive
Suite 1000
Landover, MD 20785
1 (800) 7-ASTHMA
 (1-800-727-8462)
www.aafa.org

Celiac Disease Center at
Columbia University
Harkness Pavilion
180 Fort Washington Avenue
Suite 934
New York, NY 10032

(212) 342-4529
www.celiacdiseasecenter.org

Celiac Disease Foundation
13251 Ventura Boulevard
Suite 1
Studio City, CA 91604
(818) 990-2354
www.celiac.org

Celiac Sprue Association (CSA)
PO Box 31700 Omaha, NE
 68131-0700
(877) CSA-4CSA
www.csaceliacs.org

Consortium of Food Allergy
 Research (CoFAR)
https://web.emmes.com/study/
 cofar/index.htm
(301) 251-1161
cofar@emmes.com

Culinary Institute of America
 (CIA)
www.ciachef.edu
www.ciaprochef.com/
foodallergies/about.html

Duke University Medical Center
 (CoFAR member)
Duke Children's Hospital &
 Health Center
2301 Erwin Road
Durham, NC 27710
(919) 681-3529
Duke Food Allergy Initiative:
 foodallergy@duke.edu

Duke University Information:
  http://dukehealth1.org/health_
  services/childrens_health.asp

Epi-Pen
Dey Pharma
781 Chestnut Ridge Road
Morgantown, WV 26505
1 (800) 395-3376 (main phone)
www.epipen.com

Food Allergy and Anaphylaxis
  Network (FAAN)
11781 Lee Jackson Highway
Suite 160
Fairfax, VA 22033-3309
1 (800) 929-4040
www.foodallergy.org

Food Allergy Initiative (FAI)
1414 Avenue of the Americas
Suite 1804
New York, NY 10019-2514
(212) 207-1974
www.faiusa.org

Gluten Intolerance Group® of
  North America (GIG)
31214 124th Ave. SE
Auburn, WA 98092-3667
(253) 833-6655
www.gluten.net

Johns Hopkins University
  (CoFAR member)
Pediatric Allergy/Immunology
Johns Hopkins University
600 No. Wolfe St, CMSC 1102

Baltimore, MD 21287
(410) 502-1711
www.hopkinsmedicine.org

National Association of Social
  Workers (NASW)
750 First Street, NE
Suite 700
Washington, DC 20002-4241
www.helpstartshere.org/find-a-
  social-worker
www.socialworkers.org

National Foundation for Celiac
  Awareness (NFCA)
P.O. Box 544
Ambler, PA 19002-0544
(215) 325-1306
www.celiaccentral.org

National Institute of Allergy and
  Infectious Diseases (NIAID)
Office of Communications and
  Government Relations
6610 Rockledge Drive MSC
  6612
Bethesda, MD 20892-6612
1 (866)284-4107
www.niaid.nih.gov

National Institute of Mental
  Health (NIMH) Science
  Writing, Press, and
  Dissemination Branch
6001 Executive Boulevard,
  Room 8184, MSC 9663
Bethesda, MD
  20892-9663

(866) 615-6464
www.nimh.nih.gov/index.shtml

National Jewish Health (CoFAR
  member)
CoFAR Infant Food Allergy
  Study
National Jewish Health
  Pediatric Clinical Research
1400 Jackson St. K314
Denver, CO 80206
www.nationaljewish.org

TwinJect
Shionogi Pharma, Inc.
5 Concourse Parkway
Suite 1800
Atlanta, Georgia 30328

1 (888) TWIN-JCT
www.twinject.com

University of Arkansas for
  Medical Sciences (CoFAR
  member)
Arkansas Children's Hospital
1120 Marshall Street
Suite 610
Little Rock, AR 72202
(501) 364-3749
www.uams.edu

U.S. Food and Drug
  Administration
10903 New Hampshire Avenue
Silver Spring, MD 20993
1 (888) INFO-FDA
www.fda.gov

index